Can Allergies REALLY Be ELIMINATED

Can They DO That?

BY

Robert M. Prince, M.D. and Iris W. Prince, RN

authorHOUSE®

AuthorHouse™
1663 Liberty Drive, Suite 200
Bloomington, IN 47403
www.authorhouse.com
Phone: 1-800-839-8640

First published by AuthorHouse 8/12/2008

ISBN: 978-1-4389-0988-2 (sc)

Printed in the United States of America
Bloomington, Indiana

This book is printed on acid-free paper.

DEDICATION

This book is dedicated to the memory of James Rommie Purser, the Elder and minister of the Shiloh True Light Church of Christ from 1969 until his death in 2004.

When we discussed with him how the NAET treatments might provide non-invasive, non-medication health benefits for our fellow church members, he was quite open to this innovative procedure.

He encouraged some re-structuring in the church basement itself, which became our first NAET clinic. It was here, with his encouragement and support that these services were provided freely to church members and their families over a period of several years.

TABLE OF CONTENTS

FOREWORD

I consider writing the foreword for an author who shares my interest and vision an honor; but when the author is also a friend, colleague, and supporter I consider writing the forward a pleasurable honor.

I first met Doctor Robert Prince in a class more than a decade ago. Dr. Prince, a psychiatrist, who at the time, was 66 years old and in the process of minimizing his caseload, was attending my class with no expectations. He was accompanied by his wife, Iris, and another medical professional. All of the professionals were interested in learning how to treat families and church members with nagging allergies, by using the NAET® desensitization technique.

Dr. Prince candidly admitted, during the class's introduction, the reason he was in attendance, (NAET® basic training) was because he was a doctor among a group of interested people who did not qualify to provide an independent practice (one of the requirements to receive the training.) This included his dear wife, who is a registered nurse. A born sweetheart, Dr. Prince agreed to attend because the others could not be admitted to the training unless they were accompanied by a doctor who would be their supervisor.

Even though Dr. Prince was in attendance he was still very skeptical about what I was teaching in the class. After returning home he decided to put the treatment to a vigorous test. He had suffered from an allergy to poison oak for a long time and no one could do anything about it thus far. He asked his office assistant to treat him for poison oak using the new method they had just studied. After completion of the required waiting period for the treatment to take effect, he went to the back yard and tore into a thick area of poison oak with a weed eater. At the end of his task he was amazed to see that his body did not have the usual reaction toward poison oak.

This occurrence convinced him of the powerful potential of NAET®. Since then, he has been completely devoted to NAET®. Not only did he encourage his staff to desensitize their families and church members he also decided to delve into a new practice by opening a large NAET® clinic.

Eventually he volunteered to become a trained NAET® instructor. He was the first NAET® instructor chosen to visit Europe when we decided to extend NAET® training to Europe in the year 2000. Since then he has returned to Europe to train more medical professionals.

The good words must have traveled fast because the good news is all around. His office is busy with local patients and patients who travel from different states to seek treatment from Dr. Prince and the friendly staff for various types of allergy related issues .

Without question, still to this day many undiagnosed illnesses are appearing among unsuspecting patients worldwide. The fact of the matter is that there are very few human diseases or conditions in which the ailments do not involve allergies and sensitivities, either directly or indirectly.

Potentially, one can be sensitive to anything under the sun causing various puzzling health problems. According to NAET® experience and theory, hidden sensitivities and allergies are the cause of numerous types of health problems.

For those whose lives are merely disrupted by the discomfort of the allergies or sensitivities, allopathic allergy treatments with simple antihistamine or topical remedies can bring some relief; but for more serious sufferers, long-term complete avoidance is the only solution traditional allopathic medicine can offer.

Most people finally resort to a lifetime of depriving themselves of the many things in life that would otherwise bring them joy and fulfillment. Even with avoidance, there is no guarantee that hypersensitive persons will be able to stay away from every situation and still remain reaction- free. With the progress of science and technology, the modern life-styles have changed dramatically. New chemical products, which are potential allergens for many people, are being developed every day. The quality of life has improved; but for some sensitive patients, the scientific achievements have created more nightmares.

We cannot ignore the fact that we are in the twenty first century where technology is more predominant than ever before. There is nothing wrong with the technology. In fact, modern technology has provided a better quality of life. But the allergic patient must find ways to overcome adverse reactions to chemicals and other allergens produced by the technology in order to enjoy this world. We live in diverse environments we have chosen that undoubtedly expose us to different levels of chemicals by breathing, touching and consuming. Our awareness of how sensitive we may be to our environment still does not give us immunity from chemicals we encounter along our chosen path. Our genes that came from our simple-living ancestors were not quite ready for this sudden, chemical explosion. If we had time to prepare for this situation, our genes may have adapted appropriately. Our genes are capable of naturally adapting to any situation, creating happiness and comfort in our lives, if given enough time and the right conditions. NAET has proven this claim by desensitizing thousands of people to their allergies over the past 24 years.

Health problems that arise from sensitivities and allergies tend to follow certain patterns:

Usually the allergic symptoms are reproducible by repeatedly exposing the suspected or familiar allergen, after a prolonged exposure to the allergen has occurred. However, a brief exposure can instantaneously provoke problematic symptoms (example: asthma).

Once symptoms become chronic they respond at best poorly and possibly not at all to other treatments.

Symptoms may resolve or disappear completely when the individual moves away from the triggers (going on vacation to a different state or country for a few weeks or months).

Allergic symptoms may initially begin in one area of the body and eventually may involve various organs giving rise to multiple organ symptoms – such as arthritis, asthma, attention deficit hyperactive disorders, autism, autoimmune disorders, bronchitis, chronic cough, eczema, allergies to prescription drugs, food sensitivities, learning disabilities, chronic fatigue, lupus, runny nose, itchy eyes, headache, scratchy throat, ear ache, scalp pain, mental confusion, sleepiness, palpitations of the heart, upset stomach, nausea and/or diarrhea, abdominal cramping, pain, aching joints, idiopathic pain syndrome, etc., and the list can go on.

In each of these, an allergen from the food or surroundings appears to precipitate the symptoms. The immediate trigger may be the chemical contaminants in the milk, vegetables, city water, house cleaning supplies, or cosmetics. Other irritants may be animal dander, formaldehyde in building materials, fabrics, vinyl products, chemicals in food used as additives, food colorings, processed foods, sugar products, pesticides sprayed on city trees, grasses and bushes, living near a toxic waste dump site, and heavy metal toxins. After over 24 years of allergy practice, I have learned that almost any symptom can be the result of an allergic reaction. When the allergies are detected and identified using NAET testing techniques patients have two choices: (1) Complete avoidance or (2) Elimination of the allergic reaction by desensitizing for the allergen via NAET. In most cases, allergy elimination to the desensitized allergen is permanent.

Having a successful practice for over a decade, Dr. Prince has been able to treat a wide range of commonly observed health problems with NAET with great satisfaction. He was able to collect numerous successful case studies and testimonials from satisfied patients from his office. Anyone who has tried to wrestle with an elimination or rotation diet or take antihistamines several times daily knows how frustrating that can be, not only for the patient, but also to the family and other dear ones. How wonderful it is to inform others that one doesn't have to give up allergic items or live in fear, caused by the anticipation of the next allergic reaction. That's exactly what Dr. Prince and his wife, Iris, have done in their book, "CAN ALLERGIES <u>REALLY</u> BE ELIMINATED?" In this book they have demonstrated the effectiveness of this unique allergy elimination technique by sharing a multitude of true testimonials from his practice with the reader.

Dr. Prince and his wife have tried to inform the readers about the possible encounters with known allergies and hidden ones in their daily lives. This book is very informative for people especially if they or their physicians do not know the cause of their mysterious health problems. In fact, through this valuable and informative book they are helping the readers to become smarter sleuths so that they can try to live a better life. This book is certainly an eye opener for all.

I applaud the Princes for their courage and willingness to share this valuable information with all of us. I highly recommend this book for anyone who truly wants to be set free from the captivity of chronic or acute allergies.

Devi S. Nambudripad, M.D., D.C., L.Ac., Ph.D.
The developer of NAET®
Buena Park, California

Dr. D. S. Nambudripad
6714 Beach Blvd.
Buena Park, CA 90621

Acknowledgments

First and foremost, thanks to our NAET of Carolina staff, Lesley, Selena, and Erin who are dedicated, dependable, flexible and everything we could want or need! We could not have enjoyed the past decade without them and their predecessors (and occasional fill-ins) April, Tabitha, Lauren, Beth, Mallory, Carolyn, and Amanda. You are a very special group. Many, many thanks.

Abroad our hats go off and our thanks to Jean-michel Belin for his support and tireless endeavors in bringing training to over 1200 NAET practitioners in Europe.

Our thanks to our many friends who were willing on faith to put their allergies into our hands and to learn with us. (Who do you know that would visit a psychiatrist for an allergy treatment – friend or not - or to a med-surg nurse for kinesiology?) They did, and their trust is encouraging and humbling to say the least.

To all our worldwide NAET practitioner friends, thanks for the encouragement in being a part of this pioneer movement into Wellness.

Next our thanks go to James Patrick King and to our daughter, Carol Penninger for their editorial help. They have been enormously helpful in helping us to put this book together.

Last, but certainly not least, our thanks and affections go out to Dr. Devi Nambudripad. We believe there is a God in heaven who gives insight into some of His laws of nature and physics to those who are open and willing. We believe He gives these insights to people that He knows in His foreknowledge will persistently and unselfishly make these gifts available to all mankind. It has been said that Thomas Edison failed somewhere around 10,000 times before he developed a light bulb which worked. We believe Dr. Devi was given a rare insight into the working

of the body's energy channels when she discovered **NAET**, and we applaud her for her diligence in helping to make this gift available to the whole world.

WHY WRITE ANOTHER BOOK ABOUT ALLERGIES?

1. *"Looking Back on ten years of Eliminating Allergies with NAET®"* By Robert M. Prince, MD

In the spring of 1997, several young women from our church approached my wife and me about, what seemed like at the time, a strange new way of treating allergies. They claimed a local chiropractor had been using a new drug-free approach to treat them and their families. The women pleaded for eligible church members to consider getting training to become NAET® practitioners so that this treatment would be more readily available to people in our area.

My wife, Iris, and I were somewhat skeptical when we were first introduced to this new method. The idea of pulling down on the arm and tapping on various parts of the body seemed quite peculiar compared to our traditional training. My wife had formal training as a registered nurse and I had been a psychiatrist for 35 years at that time. When we make introductory talks about NAET® in the community, we often tell that at first our intention was to investigate and debunk what seemed to be such a far-out approach. However, the earnest young women convinced us to contact the NAET® office to find out who from our church would be eligible to receive NAET® training. They informed us we could receive the training only if a doctor who was also NAET® certified would supervise them. I had hoped to sit comfortably back home in Charlotte, while they went off on this training mission, but as fate would have it, I had to accompany them. Even with our skepticism, there was still a trace of belief in our minds - that there actually maybe some credibility to this innovative approach to eliminating allergies.

We were aware of a little girl who had terribly messy diapers after she ate anything containing egg, prior to NAET treatment. The problem cleared up when she was treated with the NAET® procedure for egg mix. Due to the girl's young age it was not plausible to attribute the result to a placebo effect — since a 2 year old would most likely not respond to a placebo. Even with our mixture of skepticism and partial belief, we still hesitantly ventured out to California to learn about the NAET® process. After our first round of training, we still carried some degree of doubt since NAET® seemed to produce results almost too good to be true. When we returned home I decided to undergo treatment for a severe allergy to poison oak. My skepticism propelled me to test NAET® on an extreme personal level. Three days after receiving the treatment, I set out to prove or disprove the effectiveness of NAET® by using a weed-eater to attack an area on our property that was covered with poison oak. At the time, I had been severely allergic to poison oak for my entire life. I knew I would have a terrible rash if NAET® had not worked. Other than one tiny itching spot, which came on my neck and quickly dried up, I had no adverse reaction and I became a true believer in the power of NAET®.

In July 1997, we attended Advanced NAET® Training and our first annual NAET® Symposium in Buena Park, CA. Armed with this knowledge and our new-found enthusiasm, we began treating members of our church and their families in a free clinic at the church. Our minister was very supportive of these efforts and approved of space being set up in the basement of the church for this weekly clinic, which continued for several years.

We were especially encouraged when treating an 18-month old girl who was not standing or walking after having had surgery for clubfeet during the early weeks of her life. She was eating very poorly and showed very little interest in solid foods. She had been treated for most of the basic allergens at the church clinic, with only minimal improvement. Then one day my wife suggested that she could have been allergic to the anesthesia that she received at the time of her surgery. Two days after we treated her for anesthesia her family suddenly realized that she was standing on her own. Within a few days she was not only walking but she was running and eating an adequate amount of food. Her older brother had also been cleared of a severe allergy to milk, along with several other important food allergies. Other children treated at the church clinic, who had been plagued with stomachaches after drinking milk, were able to consume milk without adverse reactions.

Within a few months, we opened our private clinic, NAET of Carolina in Charlotte. The results continued to be very gratifying in our new clinic. The very first patient was a schoolteacher, who was having severe headaches every day she taught school. This particular year she happened to be teaching school in an older building. The previous year, in a new school building, she had no headaches. Before she came to our clinic my wife instructed her to get a sample of the air from the schoolroom where she was teaching. She was instructed to float a paper towel on a bowl of distilled water and place it on top of a cabinet near her desk and allow it to sit for two days. This allowed enough time for any toxic elements that may be in the room to settle on the moist paper towel. After 48 hours we instructed her to put the wet paper towel in a sealed jar in order to avoid contamination prior to testing. When the patient arrived at our clinic, she brought the wet paper towel in a quart jar for testing. Kinesiology (muscle testing of her arm) indicated she was definitely allergic to the substances in the jar. I used standard NAET® treatment to treat her. When she returned a week later to see her "voodoo doctor," as she called me, she said it was almost like a miracle - she had only one headache the entire week. The headache occurred on a day when there had been a lot of chalk dust stirred up in the air near her desk. After making the chalk connection she had brought a piece of chalk for testing, and she was quite allergic to it. After the chalk treatment, we heard nothing more from her about headaches.

I cautioned our practitioners that this case was much more straightforward than most headache cases. We had followed Dr. Devi Nambudripad's recommendation that allowed us to by-pass the first 10-12 basic allergens in treating this acute situation. Most people who experience chronic headaches have more complex situations and get more lasting results from clearing the basic allergens first, as recommended by Dr. Devi, the originator of NAET®.

One of my first observations while using NAET® was its amazing ability to desensitize numerous individuals to food allergies, for foods they previously had to avoid for years due to their adverse reactions. I was aware that standard allergy practices generally recognize no cure for food allergies other than avoiding the offending foods. More severe cases would be advised to keep an Epi-Pen handy in case of anaphylactic shock. We soon began seeing many individuals cleared of food allergies with great results.

A man in his early forties came in with a long history of food allergies. He would get sick if he ingested chocolates, cheese, or beer. He had been told by his doctors to stop eating a number of essential food items, including dairy products, wheat, raw vegetables, and fruits. After he was cleared of the ten basic nutrients, using the NAET® protocol, he informed us how pleasing it was to eat ice cream and fruit without adverse effects. After a few more treatments, he was able to incorporate grains and tomatoes into his diet. He was especially thrilled when he consumed pizza and beer together on a family vacation with no allergic symptoms.

A couple of years ago, we saw a middle-aged woman who had been treated with NAET® successfully four years earlier for allergies to eggs, milk, wheat, corn, nuts, and tomatoes. She had previously developed whelps when she consumed these items. On her return, she brought in a jar with cat fur and saliva, telling us that she had developed asthmatic symptoms after getting two house cats. When asked about her previous food allergies, she stated, "Oh, I can eat anything I want now." This last case, along with many others, helps to illustrate the long-lasting effects of NAET® treatments. The treatments usually yield permanent relief of food allergies, which had seriously limited their diets in the past. Is it any wonder that I spoke at Dr. Devi's annual Symposium a few years ago on the topic, <u>NAET® THE ULTIMATE TREATMENT FOR FOOD ALLERGIES?</u>

At the 2006 annual Symposium in Buena Park, CA, I gave a report on our excellent results from treating autistic children with NAET®. I did not include the case of a 5-year-old autistic boy whose family moved out of our area 4½ years ago (before he completed his treatments.) He had such severe allergies to foods, including strawberries, yogurts and several grains, that his family could not eat in the same room with him without his having a serious reaction. They had to wait for him to go to sleep before they could comfortably eat their own dinner. After treatments for most of the NAET® basic protocol, his parents reported that they were finally able to sit together for dinner - with great satisfaction that he no longer had these severe reactions. We recently called his dad to inquire about his present condition. His dad reported that he was now reading well at his third grade level, and the family now felt no need to tell anyone he had ever been classified as having been autistic. He was enjoying social activities and his dad said that he appeared perfectly normal now except for some chemical sensitivities, for which he has had some consultations and successful treatments by another NAET® practitioner. This case demonstrates how allergies are such a major factor in the exacerbation of symptoms in autistic children.

I could talk all day about other excellent results using NAET® for clients with environmental allergies, asthma, arthritis, fibromyalgia, chronic fatigue syndrome, eczema, Attention Deficit Hyperactivity Syndrome, Irritable Bowel Syndrome, and many other afflictions. But I would like to close by discussing the satisfactions that come from treating multiple members of the same family.

We have been especially encouraged that many of our patients come to us on referrals from family members who have responded well to NAET®. One case in point, a woman in her sixties who was thrilled that her NAET® treatments enabled her to eat chocolate cake while meeting with her bridge club. Previously she had to eliminate chocolate from her diet for many years. Several years later, her 7-year-old autistic grandson was referred for a series of NAET® treatments for his autism. After the treatments, he received an award for being the most improved student in his school.

An additional case of success in treating members of a single family was highlighted in our local NAET® brochure, which was published for several years with the title of "One Family's success story" as follows:

"We were especially gratified to treat a 2 1/2 year old girl who had suffered with a skin rash on her legs for most of her young life. Due to the constant itching, the child severely clawed her skin. After treatment, however, she was completely clear of the rash.

Her baby brother had a rash on his face at six weeks of age and was showing much irritability when nursing. Using a surrogate for testing and treatment, the baby was discovered to be allergic to his mother's milk. He was put on a soy formula during the 25-hour avoidance period. His mother reported that he was immediately more content when he resumed nursing. His rash disappeared within a week.

The father of the children was treated for peanut allergy and was able to eat boiled peanuts for the first time in years. When he was cleared for sugar, he was able to eat sweets without having headaches."

The members of the family just described were treated during the first weeks of our NAET® church clinic. Ten years later we have recently treated their 2-year-old son, who had eczema much like his sister's. (She is described in the above paragraph and is now 13 years old.) On the Sunday before I began writing this article, both parents approached me and my wife, Iris, outside of the church to tell us that the young son had definitely improved since his recent treatments. NAET® HAD HELPED THIS FAMILY FROM THE BEGINNING TO THE END, THROUGHOUT THE 10 YEARS WE HAD BEEN PRACTICING. NAET® HAD COME FULL CIRCLE FOR THIS FAMILY, LIKE IT CAN FOR OTHER FAMILIES IN THE FUTURE.

Note: The above is an edited version of a presentation given at the first NAET® Symposium held on European soil in France in August of 2007. Our team from NAET® of Carolina was recognized as having had the privilege of teaching the first Basic NAET® course in Europe in Holland during June 2000.

At the time of this Symposium an announcement was made that there were now over 1200 NAET® practitioners in Europe and over 9,500 worldwide.

When the book title, <u>Ca</u>n allergies **REALLY BE ELIMINATED**, first came to mind, memory immediately went back to the case of an **NAET®** practitioner in another state who was threatened by his professional board that he could lose his license for asserting that allergies could be **ELIMINATED**. The conventional teaching among allergy specialists was that there was no way to **ELIMINATE** an allergy. A number of **NAET®** practitioners wrote in support of the doctor contending that allergies **REALLY** could be **ELIMINATED**. Finally after the practitioner had been under the threat of losing his license for two years, his professional board dropped the case.

We would suggest that our readers carefully examine the evidence presented in this book before they attempt to give an answer to the question, "Can allergies **REALLY BE ELIMINATED?**"

Consider for a moment that, even though this book is primarily composed of anecdotal evidence, how many thousands of surgical operations are performed each year and are considered to be "standard medical practice." Yet many such operations have been described by doctors themselves as not having been medically necessary, and in some cases patients may have obtained better results from less invasive alternative treatments.

2. A little about the co-authors
By Iris W. Prince, RN

I believe readers would like to know why a semi-retired psychiatrist and a med-surg nurse, with more years of experience than I care to share with you — would even look seriously at a rather unusual treatment for allergies. This treatment includes aspects from several other modalities that incorporate together to become the whole of Nambudripad's Allergy Elimination Techniques.

Let me introduce myself and my husband to you, Dr. Bob Prince, MD, and his wife Iris Prince, RN. We have worked together, along with an extremely dedicated staff for the past decade. We had an interesting life before we discovered NAET®. But all of the "Standard Medicine is the only way" went out the window when we discovered NAET®, which is only a small part of what Western Medicine has overlooked and often debunked — (because it was not their idea and was also outside of their control.) Harsh words, I know, but often very true. Also the fact that oriental medicine seldom actually utilizes medicine (drugs) and then mostly herbs — takes the control away from the giant industry of medicine formulation (pill making and distribution.)

The last time I discussed any form of alternative medicine with an "educated" person, initially this person appeared interested. When I expressed myself about conglomerates that can and do try to block any progress of "competitors" in the field of health care - I watched as the eye-lids lowered, the distant look took over and heard him say — "Well, you don't want them wasting their money on Copper Bracelets."

Oh wow! How many billions of dollars are spent by consumers and their insurance companies on trying to stay well or to get well? Had I not personally witnessed a standard — simple - often used drug jump 300% in cost to the consumer in one year, I would not have been so incensed over his concern about the cost of copper bracelets. This is about control, not caring. It's a "Don't you dare think outside the box! Not my box anyway!"

Well, there are still Thomas Edisons out there who have a goal and keep trying. We as NAET® practitioners have the opportunity to work with an innovative original mind that has unearthed a unique – drug-free approach to bettering your health and we applaud her with love and respect her dedication to this enterprise.

Well, I've spouted off enough. Let us tell you the story. You might notice that my husband and I, as a team, are Yin and Yang. When we thought to write about NAET® – and its impact on <u>health care</u> – my thought was that it would be <u>so</u> confusing for someone to read a chapter by him and then another by me, when we express ourselves so differently. Well, let's say at least – I don't know how to describe myself, but the previous comments will give you the idea!

Neither of us are authors. I have jotted off a couple of brief children's books, but nothing more. He, however, is so busy thinking, that he sometimes has to talk slowly and deliberately to get it all reasoned through. You will agree about Yin/Yang. We did not undertake this of our own accord. We were urged to do this by friends whom we found hard to refuse.

3. Our approach to NCAAM

Several year after we started with NAET®, we approached the NIH (National Institutes of Health) in Washington, DC. They have a division, the National Center for Complementary and Alternative Medicine NCAAM), which offered grant money to research forms of treatment to prove or disprove their validity. We arranged with Dr. Linda Steele of the Nursing Division of UNC at Charlotte and with representatives from their Research divisions. We produced what we and they considered to be a closely monitored proposal in which we would assist in performing a double blind study that would hopefully validate the effectiveness of NAET® for allergies to corn. We were so excited over the possibility of establishing NAET® as a nationally recognized treatment for allergies. Just imagine – an alternative form of treatment that, although fairly lengthy, could be effective and validated – therefore probably (drum roll please) covered by health insurance.

NCCAM has only a few slots for Alternative Health Research and unfortunately after all our preamble of efforts including the unstinting support of the Nursing College at UNCC, we were not among the selected few. Grant money can do wonders. It can pay salaries of needed personnel while we work diligently to achieve the goal of proving what so many already know through personal experience.

A year or so later, again with excellent UNCC help, we assisted in offering an application for a more extensive double-blind study of shellfish allergies, with Dr. Steele again putting in many hours, along with assistance from the UNCC Research Department. The proposal even included the agreement of a well recognized allergy specialist at Johns Hopkins Medical Center to serve as a part-time consultant, as well as the agreement of a local Board Certified allergist to perform the Double-blind Placebo Controlled food tests. This too was turned down by NCAAM, but this time they admitted that this was research that should be done, however they said our research team was not suitably qualified to perform this project, presumably because UNCC did not have a medical school.

4. Challenge to be open to Alternative Medicine

Still we are divided into groups of "open to possibilities" and "totally closed." Many a patient has said to me, "I wish ___ _____ would try this. He has so much problem eating _____(the list is long.) How can we convince him to try this?" My answer is always, "You can't. If he's not willing to look into it after seeing your quality of life improve so much, you are wasting your breath!"

The challenge is still before us. There are actually almost endless opportunities for benefit. We must persevere patiently (he does this better than I) and work with those that are eager for help, hoping others find their way around eventually. A lot of people seem to have a problem in thinking of an electrical field connected with humans, which is one of the basic concepts upon which NAET® is founded. I ponder the fact that an electrical impulse triggers each heart beat. Also if you have ever observed an EKG or EEG, you will see the firing of electrical impulses even in sensitive brain tissue. Ah well, we cannot understand it all. I must truly say we understand only a portion of what occurs in NAET®. (Bob tells of an elderly Chinese doctor who told him that the difference between Eastern medicine and Western medicine is that we study dead tissue – hence medical students spending much of their freshman year dissecting cadavers and then pathologists perform autopsies to trace disease processes microscopically. Whereas in Eastern cultures, many have studied only live persons due to their reluctance to desecrate dead bodies – hence the discovery of acupuncture points and meridian pathways, which have helped to produce remarkable results for several thousand years.)

Being new adherents of Eastern principals we work very strictly in accord with established protocols and do not generally vary unless suggested by those who establish them. Therefore we have really had lots of successes.

We are in a "pop the pill" age and want a quick fix for whatever the problem is. However even good pills, and there are quite a few very wonderful medications, can have side effects that would astound you, and if you should be one of the unfortunate few to have them happen to you – can almost ruin the health you have left. I realize that people in dire circumstance are willing to take risks, but when your list of side effects is ended with "possible sudden death" – I believe it's time to stop and consider gentler, kinder ways to bring better health to our bodies.

The idea of preventive health is a wonderful one – right eating, clean living, with a balance of work and play, time for your family and hopefully time to grow older to see those grandchildren. I wish that it could be for all of us. It is worth working hard for, whether the steps toward it are lengthy or short.

Enough about us. Luck was with us - whenever we asked our patients for input – good or bad – stories and notes came rolling in. In the midst of all this was a patient with whom I had had several brief chats as she brought her children for treatments. She confessed that she had started a short story of her own about her travails through the very serious, allergy-related illnesses of her children. We urged her to please just send to us what she was willing to share.

Then via e-mail – in came her story, so well expressed and poignant and clear - that we decided that this should be presented to you readers – separately – in its entirety. Therefore she adds a whole new perspective to this book.

I, like so many others, have a few inconvenient allergies. So did he – but we have never been affected by the terrible problems that a great many people have. Dr. Prince was first excited by the possibility of having some hope for those who are severely limited in their diets. Current standard medicine has nothing to offer here except to stay away from it. Life-long avoidance is a difficult thing when you consider eczemas and sinusitis, vertigo, and other things that food sensitivities can cause. But the horrific warfare that mothers endure who have children with severe peanut, milk, or shellfish allergies – these can be a life or death matter with anaphylaxis as a constant threat.

Susan's Story clearly details this dilemma and is more enlightening than anything we could write.

Our goal when treating those types of life-threatening allergies is not to try for a situation where the child (or adult for that matter) might be able to enjoy seafood at leisure and as much as they might like – or even peanut butter sandwiches for severely allergic children with peanut allergies. Our goal, truly, is to desensitize a person to the point that, if there is an accidental exposure to peanuts or shellfish or whatever – that they may only be mildly inconvenienced and not hospitalized with acute anaphylaxis or worse!

You MUST read Susan's Story, a later chapter of this book. I warn you – if you are faint-hearted, the story of a mother with two severely allergic children may bring you to your knees!!

CHAPTER II

WHAT IS NAET®?

NAET® is the acronym for Nambudripad's Allergy Elimination Techniques. This process is a totally non-invasive method which can be used to treat and clear individual allergens or groups of allergens in any individual who is experiencing acute or chronic allergic manifestations. The process utilizes kinesiology, by using muscle response testing, to detect the troubling allergens the person needs to have cleared. The acupressure technique involves no needles, only tapping and/or massaging specific acupuncture points in order to desensitize specific allergens.

Unfortunately, many disease processes have hidden allergic manifestations, which are not readily detected; therefore careful detective work on the part of the patient and the NAET® practitioner is necessary in order to uncover the underlying offending agents. These allergens may manifest themselves in all degrees of severity, ranging from minor food intolerance to major anaphylactic reactions, many of which can be deadly.

1. Categories of Allergens

Allergies may be categorized into a number of different classifications. Some of the most common categories include:

Ingestants - items taken into the mouth, such as
  foods, liquids, medications, etc.
Inhalants - pollutants in the air, inhaled medications, etc.
Infectants - viruses, bacteria, etc.
Contactants - items which come in contact with the skin.

Injectants - insect stings, injected medications, etc.
Physical agents - radiation, low barometric pressure, etc.
Genetic factors - RNA, DNA, inherited traits, etc.
Molds and fungi - may also fit into ingestant or
inhalant categories.

In addition to these classifications, emotional traumas, ranging from mild to major may often play a role in aggravating almost any suspected allergic reaction.

2. History of NAET®

Dr. Devi S. Nambudripad from Buena Park, CA is the originator of this very innovative procedure. She was trained originally as a Registered Nurse, then received training as a chiropractor and acupuncturist. Then she later became a licensed Medical Doctor.

She had severe allergies to multiple foods, which limited her diet to broccoli and white rice for a period of about 3 years. After she completed acupuncture training, she found that acupuncture treatments helped to reduce the manifestations of food intolerances to the point that she was able to experiment with new food items, which expanded her nutrient intake.

Then in November of 1983, she had a very unique experience. In Dr. Devi's own words, "I was being treated by acupuncture for the relief of a severe allergic reaction to raw carrots. During the treatment, I fell asleep with the carrots still [touching] my body. After the acupuncture treatment (and a restful nap during the needling period), I woke up and experienced a unique feeling. I had never felt quite that way following other similar acupuncture treatments in the past.

I realized that I had been lying on some of the carrot. A piece was also still in my hand. I knew that some of the needles were supposed to help circulate the electrical energy and balance the body. If there is any energy blockage, the balancing process is supposed to clear it during the treatment and bring the body to a balanced state. I had studied this concept at school.

"I asked my husband, who was assisting me in the treatment process, to test me for carrots again. The carrot's energy field had interacted with my own energy field, and my brain had accepted this once deadly poison as a harmless item. The two energy fields no longer clashed. This was an amazing NEW DISCOVERY. Subsequent tests for carrots by MRT [Muscle Response Testing] confirmed that something phenomenal had happened."*

After this experience, she continued to eat carrots and found that she no longer experienced the adverse reaction. She began to hypothesize that if she received acupuncture treatment while her skin was in contact with the allergen, this would result in her no longer reacting to the particular allergen. Armed with this hypothesis she began to treat herself and members of her family to see how effective this procedure might be. She observed very positive results from this process.

Unfortunately, in the early days, numerous acupuncture needles were inserted in multiple areas of the body, making this a very cumbersome technique. Soon Dr. Devi was able to utilize her knowledge as a chiropractor to demonstrate that tapping on specific acupuncture points on the back was just as effective as using needles. This is when the preferred less invasive technique was termed as acupressure. Since no needles are required this made the method applicable to other practitioners in addition to acupuncturists.

Her chiropractic training also enabled her to use her knowledge of applied kinesiology, as exemplified by Dr. George Goodhart, a noted chiropractor, whom Dr. Devi greatly admired.

I thought it was quite interesting that one of our patients from NAET of Carolina had discovered for himself about ten years ago that allergies could be detected by holding a suspected allergen in his hand. He then had a family member pull down on his extended arm to test the strength of his arm. He said that if he held a jar of peanut butter in his hand, even his very youngest child could pull his arm down.

3. Surrogate testing

I might mention at this point, that if a person is very weak or very strong, it often becomes necessary to use a surrogate to test for allergens. Since we are dealing with pathways of electrical energy within the body, a surrogate's muscle strength may be tested while the surrogate is touching the suspected allergen and has skin-to-skin contact with the client at the same time.

In my mind I liken this example to the reaction that occurs if, hypothetically speaking, I stick my finger into an electrical outlet while simultaneously touching another person with the other hand. In this scenario I only transmit the current; I do not receive the shock. The electrical current goes right through me and shocks the other person. The same phenomenon may be imagined if several individuals are lined up, holding hands. Imagine that the person at the front end of the line sticks a key into an electrical outlet. Only the person at the opposite end of the line will feel the shock. **DO NOT TRY THIS!!**

The use of surrogates is very useful to the NAET® practitioner, because it makes possible the testing of a very young infant, a frail elderly person, or a very muscular person. Our oldest granddaughter, who was trained in NAET® about ten years ago, worked in our office for several years (before she began home-schooling her identical twin girls). One day she was checking an NFL lineman from our local professional football team. This gentleman weighed over 300 pounds, and my granddaughter was quite frail compared to his enormous build. I asked her if she had to use a surrogate to test him, and she replied, "Oh no!! When he was allergic to something his arm went right down."

When our team from NAET® of Carolina was teaching a basic NAET® course in Holland, we demonstrated to the students that the use of surrogates could successfully test for an allergen in another person even if the surrogate is allergic to the allergen. Two students were used as surrogates for each other in the demonstration. One was known to be highly allergic to egg, whereas the other was not at all allergic to eggs. When tested each was able to give an accurate test result for the other, even though their individual response was exactly the opposite.

Incidentally, when we taught the class in Holland, several of the students were kinesiologists. They told us, "We believe NAET® is the missing link for us. We knew that through our use of muscle testing, we were able to detect if a person had allergies, but we did not know how to treat them until now."

4. An overview of general procedures used in a standard NAET® treatment session

As the treatment procedure continues to evolve from Dr. Devi's successful original NAET method, she integrates the following steps in order to utilize the newer techniques so they mesh appropriately with the original techniques:

Testing and treating can be done while the patient is lying or sitting; the preferred position is lying. If the patient is pregnant, infirm or handicapped in any way, they may be treated sitting or standing. A kinesiology test is used to check the relative strengths of the muscle to be used. Our muscle of preference is in the arm and this is what we generally use. However, kinesiologists tell us that almost any muscle can be checked, and will all show weakness when exposed to an allergen.

A surrogate can easily be used if there is a problem of strength, too much or too little, or of general accessibility (Example: a hyperactive or autistic child may be constantly moving).

There are techniques available to promote "balance" of the body's polarities if they are in a state of imbalance (underhydration, stress from strenuous exercise, or extreme weakness from illness.) There are temporary balancing procedures that produce a normal state long enough to be evaluated and treated.

A brief word about Yin/Yang balance; in Chinese medicine, the term "Yang" stands for strength and "Yin" for weakness. But that is a great over-simplification. Yang stands for light, Yin stands for darkness, Yang for male, Yin for female, Yang active, Yin passive, etc. Yet they are none of these things. They are opposites of each quality. A client once responded, "Oh, Yang is good, Yin is bad!" That is not correct. Good and bad are value judgments and imply desirable or undesirable. The secret of Yin and Yang is the desirability of a balance between the two. Each has its job and should harmoniously balance the other to perform well.

Therefore, a few moments must be taken at the beginning of each treatment to check for and to institute a balance in polarity if it is not present. A general testing of muscle strength is also done by touching various organ points on the body. If weakness is detected, the organ may be balanced by brief gentle massage of the examiner's fingertips over the organ point. This has taken much longer to explain than it would to perform.

After the balancing procedures have been done, a suspected allergen is placed in the client's hand. Allergies may be detected on one or more of these three levels: (A) Physical (Structural), (B). Nutritional (Chemical) or (C) the Emotional levels.

Muscle strength is also tested by touching the organ points again. Several organ points usually will be weak in the presence of the allergen. (No massaging is done at this time; however, any weaknesses should be cleared by the subsequent treatment.)

The actual treatment does not take very long, and is performed by tapping on appropriate points along specific acupuncture meridians located on the back.

After treatment is completed, the client continues to hold the allergen while the Physical, Nutritional and Emotional levels are tested again. Occasionally we find the allergen will clear on levels A and B, but will not clear on level C (the emotional level). This requires special treatment for the emotional level. Retesting of the muscle strength over the organ points is performed when necessary. If any weakness is still present, the client is treated again until all weaknesses are cleared.

Generally after the treatment is completed, we use a special "gate closing" procedure to rebalance the body – there are exceptions to this, one case in point being when treating very young children.

This brief procedure is accomplished with gentle fingertip massage or a light vibrator massage on 6 to 10 of the acupuncture points over the outer perimeter of the body. The term "gate closure" is a derivative of the oriental idea of "gates" to the body's energy, otherwise known as meridian pathways.

At the end of the treatment the client, who is still in contact with the allergen, will sit quietly for 15 to 20 minutes without any other stimulation – no reading, watching TV, no crossing arms or legs, etc. The body should be linear at this time, mirroring the energy flow that is encouraged. Absolutely no leg crossing or arms crossing across the chest is allowed during this fragile time. This time of stillness is pertinent because the body is processing new energy information. Often clients use this time to relax in a meditative state.

However, in our clinic this "holding, relaxing area" is in a very large room and we find that often socially minded people can't resist the urge for a good chat. "How long have you been coming here?" "Has it helped?" "What are you being treated for?" The last question occasionally evokes feelings of much embarrassment, due to the numerous personal items that we find in ailing patients after the basics are completed. We often encourage clients to avoid asking questions that could potentially cause embarrassment.

A word about BBF, a balancing treatment devised by Dr. Devi several years ago. We now use BBF routinely as the very first step of the treatment protocol. Before implementing BBF we began with the step dealing with nutrients. We have found when we use BBF as the first treatment it greatly facilitates the ease with which all the following treatments respond.

Any way, after all the above has been completed, one more arm check is done before the patient is free to leave with what some think of as the hard part still to come. The PATIENT IS REQUIRED TO STRICTLY AVOID THE ITEM FOR WHICH HE OR SHE WAS TREATED. In the case of foods, the patient must avoid anything containing the nutrients in it, and often times must refrain from touching the item. This painstaking process only lasts for a 25-hour period – which is the amount of time required for energy to pass through the meridian system. This can be difficult, but if it is not carried out carefully, the client may not pass on retest at the time of the next visit. Not to mention a failed treatment can make a person feel pretty rotten.

After returning to the clinic at any time after 25 hours, there is a brief rechecking procedure that tests the effectiveness of the previous treatment. If all is clear, we proceed to the next item.

Let us say a few words about the necessity of following the protocol of treatments:

The protocol usually starts with simple nutrients. The egg mix includes egg white, egg yolk, chicken, feathers, and tetracycline (which is fed to chickens and then we get exposed to it.) Unless a person is extremely allergic to one of the individual components, these can usually be treated at the same time.

Then other nutrients are addressed, such as calcium mix, B-complex mix, and others, which are building blocks in nutrient strength. Only rarely do we vary from this protocol when the body indicates a need to briefly treat an out-of-order item.

Here again there are occasional exceptions, such as a quick fix for an acute temporary situation – which also has a specific protocol.

We have also found that if treatments are done in the prescribed order – when we reach a particularly worrisome agent for that person – their reaction is already weakened – and usually clears easily. Whereas, if we try to jump to a "big" bothersome item – treatment does not go as well.

We remember at our very first training session, we were specifically cautioned to check and treat each other for the first protocol items and to avoid serious allergens. One of the ladies in the practice session requested that her partner check and treat her for horse dander because she felt she "probably was allergic to it." Later she admitted that she noticed a shortness of breath when in the presence of horses. THIS WAS NOT A GOOD IDEA! She experienced an intense reaction to the treatment and we had the golden opportunity to see the techniques used to revive a person who had completely passed out. Needless to say it is better to avoid this shortcut that had such serious consequences!

The reader can see that NAET® is not a quick fix, but it is a very methodical way of tracking down significant allergies in order to desensitize them. Usually one item at a time is desensitized, or one group of items at a time (such as B-complex vitamins where approximately 16 B vitamins are desensitized at one time.)

Occasionally a person who has a specific symptom which can be traced back to one or two specific allergens may get dramatic improvement in one or two treatments. This was discussed in the previous chapter about a schoolteacher who experienced headaches every day she taught school. She reported great improvement after being cleared from a sample of air from her schoolroom and a sample of chalk.

5. A letter from the mother of a son with multiple food allergies, describing the relief obtained after NAET® treatments

June 29.2008

Dr. Prince

I wanted to respond to your e-mail in regards to how NAET has helped Nathan in hopes that his story will help many other children. Prior to visiting your office we had been though a seven year battle trying to find help for Nathan who had been diagnosed with ADHD, OCD, sensory integration, visual processing disorder, developmental delays, eczema, sleep problems, and a host of other labels. We spent those seven long years trying almost everything: occupational therapy, physical therapy, speech therapy, music therapy, behavioral modification, bio-feed back, brain wave scans, three different neurologists, every medication ever recommended, and countless therapists.

We even flew to Dallas, Texas to have a doctor evaluate Nathan with numerous tests. She took nine tubes of blood, conducted food and inhalant allergy testing, and many other things to discover he was suffering from acute food allergies, vitamin deficiencies, hypoglycemia and of course was developmentally delayed due to years of struggling with all of the above.

There were early signs that Nathan had food allergies but none of the multiple pediatricians recognized it nor did we as parents know the symptoms. As an infant, he would have projectile vomiting, had acute ear infections and eczema. He had tubes put in his ears at 18 months old after ten ear infections and one that almost lead to a perforated ear drum. As concerned parents, we kept asking the doctors what was going on with our son but no one could give us any answers.

By the time he started preschool at age four, we knew he was not developing as quickly as other children. His preschool teacher recommended he not attend kindergarten but be enrolled in a transitional program to give him more time to develop. We listened but went on to seek a full evaluation from a local psychologist and neurologist. Thus, all of the above mentioned labels and diagnosis.

After years of struggling to find answers for this child we began to look into alternative methods. The doctor in Texas encouraged us to take Nathan off of all medications and try a food elimination diet along with vitamin supplements. The results were amazing but he often felt deprived by not being allowed to have any wheat, gluten, dairy, casein, eggs, etc. His diet was extremely limiting and frustrating at times.

A friend at church who has a daughter with Autism told us about NAET and how Dr. Prince had helped her daughter overcome food allergies similar to Nathan's. She warned us that the treatment was strange and sometimes referred to as "Voo-Doo." My husband and I had worked as Sunday school teachers with this child and knew her symptoms well. The mom spoke so highly of Dr. Prince and the program that we felt it was worth a try.

Nathan has been though about 26 treatments and is doing well. In the past, he was not able to take part in communion at church due to the wheat crackers but recently he has been able to participate without adverse reactions. Once while at school, he had a reaction to an apple even though he did not eat it but simply came in contact with it. He was treated for apple with NAET a couple times and can now eat foods containing apple.

One of his main indicators of an allergy reaction would be red-hot ears, hyperactivity or extreme fatigue and sometimes a burning throat. We are thrilled that he has been medication free for a year and we do not see signs of those old labels.

He recently turned 13 years old and has grown about 2 inches in last few months. Many friends and relatives have remarked how much different Nathan is now. He is happier, more out-going, growing and eating like crazy.

We want to encourage people to take a step of faith and look beyond traditional medical approaches in their search for answers. We truly believe God worked a miracle in our son's life by revealing food allergies as the underlying issue causing his symptoms. We are eternally grateful for what NAET has done for Nathan and look forward to continued success.

Blessings,
Angela and Ben Williams

Chapter III

EMOTIONAL ASPECTS OF ALLERGIES

1. General Observations of emotions provoked by allergies or vice-versa

Three divisions of allergy that are treated by using NAET® are physical, physiological, and emotional. Most people are aware of the physical reaction to allergies. Others who are affected by physiological problems are aware of the nutritional or chemical allergens – being affected by them or having acquaintances who must suffer the discomforts of them.

However few of us will even acknowledge the presence of emotional allergic reactions (or the ability of our bodies to react strongly in a negative way to something due to an emotional sensitivity.) This emotional sensitivity and its profound reaction is the component I will address here. We are all familiar with the unnerving feelings we can experience when reminded of a very disturbing occurrence. Upon passing the spot on a road where we had observed a shocking accident occur - we will often even feel a shiver or a profound feeling of unease – long after the time of the initial fear and alarm have passed. Gradually, this reminder of our original unease will diminish until much later. We may only feel a small sense of disquiet.

Our ways of dealing with emotional sensitivities are not simple. Often, after the original trauma, the event and its feelings are completely forgotten or purposely repressed. We go on completely unaware that emotionally the memory may be significant enough to be stored away from our conscious thoughts.

It may later resurface as a slight withdrawing when exposed to the causative agent or condition. It can, however, be expressed by a strong reaction, physical or emotional when exposed to the thought (panic attack), physical sensation or visual stimulation (phobias and generalized fear.)

I believe our emotional reactions are most commonly under-rated and often dismissed by others, with a "Just get-over-it" attitude. If emotions were easily controlled consciously, then we would all truly get over it and go on with our lives. However emotions are a powerful governing force to be dealt with - and without some assistance in relieving these strong feelings, when they are negative, they can, and often do, proceed to control your lives. As in the case of agoraphobia, claustrophobia, etc., they can also affect the lives of those around us.

I am reminded of a professional legal secretary who would invite me to lunch and then ask me to park, come into her building, ride up to the 8th floor and "pick her up." She would never board the elevator alone – but at time to leave for the day would wait for someone else to leave. Then she would quickly catch up to them and ride down the elevator when they did. Coming in early in the AM, she always had plenty of company. Lunch time was a high anxiety time for her until she learned someone else was going out. Our phobias, understood or not, can control us and others.

Pavlov's experiment with dogs and training them to salivate at a sound – a process which led to the theory of "conditioned response," is commonly true of our emotions, also. The problem is, as I see it, we are often unaware of what the connections are, or how to undo them.

Occasionally there are deeper undertones to allergies which may involve stored emotions, which may prevent their easy clearing. An experienced NAET® practitioner will know how to recognize and treat those fears.

On a training trip to Holland in 2000, we were demonstrating the NAET® procedures to novice NAET® trainees. Usually this begins with the basic protein: egg mix. Each student was giving and later receiving, a treatment for this basic nutrient, if they were found to be sensitive to it or to one of its component parts (egg yolk, egg white, chicken, feathers, and tetracycline which is frequently fed to chickens.)

We were teaching and observing for responses when I became aware of sobbing at the end of the room. I went immediately to the table and questioned both the treater and "treatee." Both trainees were as amazed as I was. The lady being treated could not believe she had any trouble with egg mix. She said she always loved eating egg salad sandwiches and always fixed one for herself when she was young and anything upset her.

She had taken in a lot of comfort with her sandwiches, but also must have kept inside a lot of unhappiness. This demonstrates a concept about "eating your allergies" that I believe is very true. Our bodies may confuse our low emotional state as being due to what we are eating at the time. It is possible we often crave the things we are sensitive to. We may have used them as "comfort foods" when under stress, which our bodies decided not to accept without strong resistance. Adverse reactions which might result include stomach ache, colitis, indigestion, rash, etc. The wonderful part is, by consciously bringing these things to focus, they can be successfully treated.

2. Self-treatments for Emotions

Generally, it is better to treat and clear emotional upsets as they occur. Emotions do not just go away, but as a form of energy may resurface unexpectedly at a later time and as a totally unexpected response.

Major emotional issues require the guidance and assistance of a professional who is competent to manage not only their clearing, but the aftermath following the treatment. Major emotional problems are a very real health issue and may cause many days of lost work productivity every year.

On a more personal level – money and lost wages may be the least of the repercussions from emotional upheavals, and may extend into major mental illnesses, such as depression, compulsive disorders or suicides. Unresolved serious emotional issues most surely result in a miserable existence. The cost to the individual cannot be determined with any accuracy.

There is a tendency in the practice of allopathic medicine to completely separate the problems of emotional disorders and those of physical ones, except when stressful physical illnesses produce accompanying emotional issues. Then they are grudgingly acknowledged and in a tactful, but minimizing way. Valium and other subsequently favored mood altering relaxers, sleep aids, and stress busters (Aptiva, Xanax, Lunesta, etc.) are brought into play.

I am not negating their value in acute stress, but the habit-forming potential of this type of medical support is profound, and a real problem for numbers of patients who naively continue the use of these drugs beyond a brief period of time.

To be able to take control of minor emotional issues and their disturbing symptoms, the NAET® Emotional Self-treatment is generally as follows:

1. Find a quiet relaxing place, alone, to focus on the issue you want to resolve. (Where quiet is preferable, I have found myself pulled over beside the road, tapping away at my emotional points if I have just encountered a harried driving experience.)

2. Try to visualize the unsettling experience itself. This is probably easier with your eyes closed. Contact points #1 and #2 as follows: (a) Place your right three fingers on Point #1 and your left three fingers on Point #2. Keep

in contact with both points during the procedure. (See diagram of self-help points below.)

3.Then tap with the right finger tips on Point #1 while reliving the memory of the incident for about 30-60 seconds.

4.Then tap with the left finger-tips on Point #2 for 30–60 seconds while thinking positive or pleasant thoughts related to the incident. It is important to maintain contact with both points during the procedure.

Diagram of Self Help points

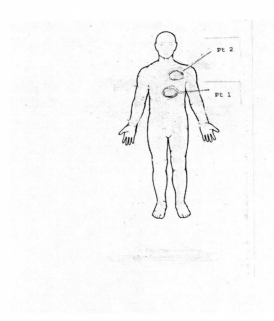

If it is easier to massage points rather than to tap them, you may massage CLOCKWISE for 30-60 seconds on each point.

It is surprising how you can replace a strong negative emotion with a positive one – and how effective this can be in re-establishing an emotional balance to yourself.

5. Letter from patient treated with NAET for fear flying; muscle pain and headaches

March 2003

Dear Dr. Prince

As you know, NAET is responsible for curing me of my food and environmental allergies, completely removing the muscle pain and debilitating headaches from which I suffered for years. A recent experience convinced me NAET has also eliminated my long standing fear of flying.

I was on board a plane at the Charlotte airport where we were taxiing for take off. Suddenly, the plane stopped and we saw smoke rising near the end of the runway. The Captain informed us of the crash of a commuter plane just taking off. He then moved the plane to the side of the taxiway. From out my window, I observed the firefighting and unsuccessful rescue efforts. Although I presumed we would return to the airport, after about an hour we took off.

Before my NAET treatment, I was often very anxious about flying even in the best of conditions. After what I witnessed, my mind would have churned with the terrible possibilities that could happen to me. Instead, while I felt sadness at the deaths of the passengers, I had a calm, detached feeling throughout the experience. I didn't even realize how well I had handled the situation until I was on the ground at my destination.

NAET is a wonderful life-changing treatment. I'm very thankful to Dr. Nambudripad, you and your wonderful staff for helping to restore my life to a state of excellent health and now for making travel a pleasure.

Gratefully,

John Brock

Note: John describes above the treatment he got for his fear of flying, which consisted of his thinking of his considerable fear while being given an emotional treatment, tapping on his back with the NAET protocol while he concentrated on these thoughts.

Pam and John have kept in touch with us by e-mail from time to time. His relief from the fear of flying is even more significant when we consider he has a very responsible job in Alabama, which entailed his making a business trip (including a 20 hour flight to South Africa) in the spring of 2008, during which time he went on several safaris into the jungle. Pam let us know he simply would not have gone 10 years ago.

Several months earlier, their loyalty to NAET was shown when they were listening to Dr. Oz's XM radio program at a time when he was interviewing Dr. Jacob Teitelbaum, whom we all know is well respected as an authority on Fibromyalgia and Chronic Fatigue Syndrome and as being married to an NAET practitioner. They sent us an e-mail, telling how they stood up and cheered when they heard a positive reference about NAET. Pam informed us she has written Dr. Oz's producers several times recommending Dr. Devi be interviewed on Dr. Oz's program. RMP

Remarks from Pam An unexpected bonus

March 2008

"I came to NAET without special allergies - that I knew of. I remember after the basic 10, I didn't have any more car sickness, in fact I could actually read in the car. I wouldn't have thought of that as an allergy so it wasn't something I tracked. I just noticed later that riding in the mountains was no longer a bother."

Pam Brock formerly from Hickory NC, now in Huntsville, Alabama.

Chapter IV

SUSAN'S STORY
by Susan Patnaik

"In health there is freedom. Health is the first of all liberties."
- Henri Frederic Amiel

It was my daughter Natalie's first birthday. The lights dimmed, a hush fell over the room and cameras popped up here and there as mommy and daddy led their princess through a crowd of guests to the drum-roll moment, the cutting of her picture perfect cake - a confection of epic proportions, a multi-layer chocolate creation slathered with white butter-cream frosting and latticed with mint green leaves and pastel flowers of pink, yellow and blue. Hidden inside was the final added touch, the little something extra, the piece de resistance: hazelnut cream filling.

Dressed in a summer pinafore the color of daffodils with her wispy black hair slowly pulling loose from what had been a flawless ponytail, Natalie stared sideways at the crowd over the top of the sugary monument. Her proud father took his baby's hand in his and together they cut the first piece. The crowd cheered. "Give the birthday girl the first piece!"

After just one bite Natalie refused to take another, even as children all around her buried their faces in a feeding frenzy of cake and icing. *Maybe my child just has more sense than the rest of them,* I thought to myself trying to brush aside her behavior. Still, as most mothers do, I longed for Natalie to grant me the satisfaction of knowing I had gotten something right, splendidly right.

By the growing look of horror on her face, a little icing still smeared in the corners of her mouth, it soon became obvious *splendidly right* was not going to be my fate that day. Within minutes her face morphed from a perfection of smooth alabaster to a grotesque swelling of splotchy, red hives. *What is that?* My mind turned on itself in a form of mommy interrogation that had become second nature after a challenging year of baby mysteries. *Exhaustion? Heat rash?* It was June, after all. *Or could something have spilled on Natalie?* The detective dug deeper with questions. *Maybe it will go away,* I reasoned – hoped rather - turning my attention back to the guests. "Who would like some cake? Can I get you some cake?" I carried on.

Moms everywhere know "it" – whatever "it" is – never goes away that easily. As much as we would like to turn our back on those odd occurrences that happen now and then with our children and tell ourselves they probably don't matter much in the grand scheme of things, we cannot. At least we cannot for very long. There always remains a nagging little voice inside of us – sometimes waking us up in the middle of the night – challenging us to look deeper, listen more closely, and even fly straight into the face of conventional wisdom if need be in order to understand our children's needs.

But on Natalie's birthday, it was not that voice – the voice of motherly wisdom - that cried out to me. That voice was still relatively weak at the time and could easily be drowned out by the distractions of the party. No, it was Natalie's voice that knew it had to speak up and it was Natalie's voice that followed me through the crowd as I tried to escape, filling the room with a nagging cry, not one too high nor too loud but one that was persistent. Not a cry that said *I'm tired* or *I'm hungry* or *someone took my toy away.* Rather a cry that said *Help me!*

Until that moment, Natalie – a people person since birth - had been the perfect hostess, bouncing from guest to guest flattering her admirers with high-voltage smiles and laughter and hugs and kisses. She was not one to whine or blubber-on over nonsense, especially in the presence of a captive and generous audience. I had never witnessed a more sudden mood swing in Natalie. It was sunshine to thunderstorms in a matter of minutes, no warning and no explanation.

"Please stop crying, Natalie" I knelt down next to her and begged, feeling a headache coming on and fearing the guests were about to leave. "Don't you want some cake? Maybe that will make you feel better." The wailing spiked a pitch. "Okay. No cake."

Finally, I heard someone call out from the crowd. It was another mother – one with older children and more experience than myself. "Looks like she's having an allergic reaction," she said.

"An allergic reaction? To what?" I challenged the suggestion.

"The birthday cake I would think," came the answer.

The birthday cake? That's strange! I had never heard of such a thing.

But at that point I was willing to consider anything. I followed the mother's advice and gave Natalie some Benedryl. I did not call a doctor. I did not call an ambulance. In fact, my husband and I were so oblivious to the dangerous nature of Natalie's reaction that we carried on with picture taking despite Natalie's disfigured face.

"Smile Natalie!" we said as we tried to recover the spirit of the party.

A few months and a number of blood tests later, I received the official verdict on my super-deluxe birthday cake.

"Your daughter is severely allergic to nuts, Mrs. Patnaik. What kind of cream did you say was in the cake ... hazelnut?" asked the doctor.

"Yes, that's right," I confessed.

We had sought out a well-respected pediatric allergist widely known from New York City to New Haven, an expert the major networks turned to when their morning talk shows wanted to shed light on the growing problem of food allergies among young children.

By this time Natalie had grown into a 15-month-old bundle of spunk who did not take kindly to her stay-at-home mother sharing even a smidgen of attention with some strange man in a lab coat. And she had her own ways of neutralizing the threat: a few cotton balls in the mouth, a quick yank on the stethoscope, vicious kicking of the examination table, and when all that failed, a quick dash out the door and down the hallway.

"Well, I'm looking here at the lab report," the doctor maintained his composure obviously accustomed to the volatile antics of his younger patients. "Natalie's IgE test result for hazelnut was 1.50. That means her immune reaction to hazelnuts falls within Class 3 or the Moderate Positive range.

Let's see now, I'm thinking. *IgE ... 1.50 ... Class 3 ... okay, how am I going to remember all this?* I stick my hands in my purse searching for pen and paper while nervously checking around for Natalie. I feel a sweat coming on. *It's chemistry class all over again. That was my only C in high school.*

The doctor continued on in lecture mode, "A result of Class 3 alone does not necessarily indicate a severe allergy. It's actually a somewhat mid-range test result with Class 1 being Very Low Positive and Class 6 — the highest class - being Extremely High Positive. But when you combine it with the reaction your daughter experienced, a Class 3 result is significant in that it reinforces out conclusion. She is allergic - severely allergic - to hazelnuts."

"So she should never eat a hazelnut again," I said ready to grab Natalie and wrap things up. "I think we can manage that."

"Now let's look at the other results, Mrs. Patnaik. There are a few other foods Natalie should avoid. She's a Class 4 – High Positive – on almonds, peanuts and egg white. Has she ever been exposed to those foods?" the doctor sucked me back in.

"No almonds and no peanuts," I said confidently, "but eggs certainly. She likes scrambled eggs." I looked over at her as she flashed me her *I Love You* smile. "She doesn't eat them all the time, but she's definitely eaten eggs with no reaction, nothing to warrant a High Positive score on eggs," I tried to reason, feeling myself starting to sink into intellectual quick sand.

"Well, given your child's test results and the family history," he searched up and down Natalie's chart. "Natalie's father is allergic to eggs . . . I believe you indicated that in the family history," the doctor looked to me for confirmation.

"Yes," I confess again.

"That confirms it. Let's take her off eggs for now. And limit milk and soy products." The doctor checked the report again. "She's a Class 2 on those. At her age a child like Natalie, one who is showing allergic sensitivities, should avoid common food allergens. Strict avoidance is the best way to give her immune system a chance to grow and strengthen. The last thing you want is a Class 2 result to develop into a Class 3 or Class 4. Which brings me to Natalie's Class 4 result for peanuts and almonds."

Lord help me! When is this going to be over? No nuts, no eggs, no milk products . . . that means cheese, yogurt, butter . . . no soy products . . . actually we don't eat any soy products. I can live with that one. What does that leave us with, bread? But maybe the bread we eat is made with eggs. *Guess I'll have to check that. Where's Natalie? Oh, there she is.* "Stop it!" I say reflexively with my eyes, knowing it will apply somehow.

"The peanut allergy is the most alarming. Natalie's antibody level was 4.15 for peanuts. That qualifies as Class 4 – High Positive. With a result like that she is at risk for anaphylaxis," the doctor carried on in expert mode.

"Ana-what?" I managed to interject. By this time Natalie could have wandered off to the nurses' station and I don't think I would have noticed.

"Ana...phyl...axis," the doctor continued with his "Allergic reactions occur when...... benign substance like food... immune response... mild symptoms, sneezing, wheezing, itching...anaphylaxis, sudden allergic reaction, whole body... cardiovascular system, drop in blood pressure, loss of consciousness, total shock... potentially resulting in death."

What did he say? Ana-what? I still couldn't swallow that word and I never did find a pencil and who knows what hallway Natalie wandered down. My heart began to race. My breathing became shallow. Time stood still for a moment as I tried to collect my thoughts. It was as if I was having my own mini-reaction to the word anaphylaxis itself. The rest of the doctor's explanation, his careful, detailed description, evaporated somewhere between "benign substance" and "loss of consciousness." I reassured myself I could look it up some other time, if it became necessary. All I really wanted at that point was to bust out of that 10x8 foot room, grab my baby, go home and take a nap.

Like most first-time mothers, I was still struggling up the steep learning curve of motherhood and honestly did not have room in my brain for a word like "anaphylaxis" – let alone room in my heart for a concept like "sudden allergic reaction potentially resulting in death." I only knew what I had witnessed firsthand: after one small bite of hazelnut cream Natalie's face had broken out in hives and she had erupted in tears. Then everything had been brought back to normal with antihistamine. But her blood pressure? Her heart rate? Her respiratory system? There was no way to assess those vital signs after the fact. Why jump to the conclusion she had been near death? Besides, it was easier to embrace the positive and believe Natalie's condition to be on the less severe side. Of course, to be safe, we would certainly follow our doctor's recommended food restrictions – for the time being – until Natalie outgrew her sensitivities. And at that point I felt incapable of anything other than embracing that as a certainty.

Natalie was a Y2K baby and an NYC baby as well. She had been born in the year 2000 in New York City; confetti from the turn of the millennium celebration was probably still floating in the air in June when she was born. It was a time when optimism and jubilance rang in the streets as the bull market bolted onward and upward and advancements in technology held out the promise of a future so bright it was hard to ponder without bringing on vertigo. Natalie entered the world with spirits all around her soaring to new heights only to plummet to new depths in 2001 with the terrorist attacks in September.

It was in this environment – this emotional, political and spiritual whirlwind – that I was introduced for the first time to the concept of life threatening food allergies and the tongue twisting word – anaphylaxis. If I was slow to embrace the cause of the Food Allergy Mom it could also be that one's psyche can only swallow so much at one time. Suicide madmen killing our friends and neighbors - that brought all of us to our knees. Deadly proteins disguised as food that could steal my child away from me in as little as one bite – that one knocked me on down to the ground. It would take time and energy to find my footing in this strange new world.

It helped that we no longer lived in Manhattan. A few weeks before Natalie was born, we had nested in a small town in Connecticut, a commuting town. It was a Norman Rockwell look-alike, a vista one could easily imagine on a vintage sampler, embroidered here and there with rolling hills, old stone walls, burbling streams and winding roads – roads with names like Deer Run, Canterbury and Cherry Lane. There was even a Lover's Lane twisting and turning through the forested terrain, leading to a hidden meadow and spring water pond where the children would swim and the town folk gathered each year to celebrate the 4th of July. Around six every evening a train would chug through town, stop at the local station and return the commuters from the city, mostly young father's who were often greeted by children jumping from their mothers' arms with a squeal and a cheer, "Daddy's home!" Natalie and I were often among the mix.

But cheering and all other expressions of joy came to a full stop on September 11th. Several daddies and I believe at least one mommy never came back into town on the train which had carried them to work that morning. Mothers all over the country held their children closer than ever as they pondered the new dangers lurking in the world and the question that left them pacing back and forth at night unable to sleep: what in the world was a mother to do?

My only solace was to be found in the daily rituals of mothering: bathing and dressing Natalie, brushing her first few teeth, singing nursery rhymes and strolling around town together watching the leaves slowly release their hold on life and then eventually fall and gather at our feet. With the arrival of Halloween we finally saw smiles again. Natalie delighted everyone waddling around as Charlie Chaplin with her smoky eyes and pitch black hair curled in a mop on her head and a stubby mustache penciled in with my eyeliner.

It was the first time I can remember thinking about nuts and peanuts again. I was already following the doctor's recommended dietary restrictions when preparing Natalie's food. For the time being it was not too complicated. Her favorite foods were avocados, liverwurst, broccoli, fig newtons, rice and crackers. Cow's milk and soy milk had been restricted by the doctor, so Natalie was drinking rice milk, a sugary, watered-down milk concoction made from fermented brown rice. To everyone's relief, she loved it.

The danger of nuts and peanuts, however, seemed remote until I saw peanut M&M's and chocolate almond kisses flying threw the air at us as we knocked on door after door in our apartment complex. "Stop throwing nuts at us!" I wanted to shout. Instead, I politely declined most of the candy we were offered and cut the circuit short.

We found a safe haven that night in the loving home of close friends in the complex, a family of five – mother, father, teenage daughter, preteen son, and Yorkshire terrier – all of whom loved and doted on Natalie, watching her occasionally if I needed to run errands or take a mommy break. The mother and I had grown into good friends in the last year, bonding over the struggles of motherhood, hers a little different from mine but nonetheless complicated and in need of a sympathetic ear. She - having raised two happy, healthy, well-adjusted children – had become a role model and mentor for me, a rare find for a new mother.

She was one of the few people I had told about Natalie's food allergies. I remember carefully checking for her reaction as I told her about what for me was a previously unheard of condition. If I thought it was preposterous, what would others think when I told them? Would they write me off as some kind of overprotective mother trying to shield her child from every possible germ in the world? I remember talking about the condition as if it was completely hypothetical, something I wasn't convinced of yet, but would be watching out for. But

I was always made it clear that Natalie shouldn't be given any nuts of any kind.

My friend listened sympathetically. She told her husband and children. They looked puzzled but concerned. It was as if a new disability had been declared – the "I can't eat peanut butter and jelly sandwiches" disability. I might as well have told them Natalie was allergic to childhood. Poor Natalie!

My dear friends were careful not to give Natalie peanut butter. That seemed a fairly obvious violation of her dietary restrictions. But their apartment – home to two adolescent kids – was full of snacks of all kinds, none of which I ever thought to question.

Not long after that night of trick-or-treating, I dropped Natalie off for an afternoon with our friends. As soon as they opened the door, Natalie marched in and made herself at home in the family where there was never a dull moment, a welcome contrast to the overly organized and sedate environment of our own apartment. "Bye Natalie!" I must have called after her. I doubt there was a response. There was always fun to be had with the older kids and she never wasted a minute getting down to business. It was certainly better than having her cling to my leg refusing to let me leave her - even if I did feel a little forgotten.

Upon my return, Natalie never failed to make up for her previous dismissals with hugs and kisses and huge smiles. But that day when I came back to pick her up she was a mess, wailing and shrieking as if she was on fire. She looked to me, her mother, the one person who was supposed to be able to speak her language, and she let me have it, flailing her arms about and demanding a solution to her distress. My friend and her children had been holding her for over an hour trying to calm her tantrum with no success. They shrugged, saying her behavior was all very mysterious, but they did admit to having allowed her to take a bite of a peanut butter cookie. "It was just one bite," they said. "We realized it just as she put it in her mouth. You don't think one bite could be dangerous do you?"

No, I really didn't and I could understand their disbelief. But at that point I had a fire to put out – if only I could find it. I swept Natalie up in my arms and raced back to our apartment.

"Natalie, calm down. Talk to me. Tell me what hurts. Where? What are you feeling?" I pleaded all the way home. There wasn't a tummy ache, a diaper rash, or a teething gum I hadn't been able to soothe with mommy comfort – a special combination of rocking and humming and dim lights and soft blankets and a little whispering. Nothing had defied my secret talents.

Nothing until that night. Natalie just wailed and wailed. She reminded me of a fire alarm with its incessant blaring, calling everyone to action. But what was to be done? She obviously had no trouble breathing. I went to change her diaper, looking for clues more than anything else. As I pulled up her dress I saw her belly was covered in hives. I gasped. *What did the doctor say to do again?*

Within five minutes Natalie and I were being whisked away in an ambulance to the emergency room.

Natalie's first few strange reactions to food marked the beginning of a journey . . . a journey which has shaped my life far more dramatically than I care to reflect upon generally. But when examined, yes, the impact has been undeniably great. The word anaphylaxis did not exist for me before the age of 34. Before that word introduced itself to me, allergies made people sneeze, not die. Before that word joined my family, food could do nothing worse to you than pack on a few pounds.

Before that word threatened to steal my child, a cracker was a snack not poison in disguise.

Motherhood, in and of itself, is a journey, one I had visualized as challenging in a predictable sort of way and one for which I felt I was prepared. The presumed inviolability of my well-laid plans made it difficult at first to find any value in the intrusion of anaphylaxis into my more romantic version of motherhood. Although the experience has turned out to be quite different from the one I envisioned, little by little as the hidden blessings have begun to reveal themselves I have come to embrace the journey as my own.

I am now the mother of two children who have suffered from food allergies, my daughter Natalie and my son Harris. Both Natalie and Harris have experienced and survived a number of food-related anaphylactic reactions. Natalie's reactions were linked to peanuts and tree nuts whereas Harris's reactions were caused mostly by milk proteins but at least one was linked to nuts.

With all due respect to our pediatric allergist and his gentle, painstaking descriptions, no text-book explanation of anaphylaxis can evoke an understanding that comes close to the actual experience. If you've ever lived through an earthquake I imagine you could say the same thing. Words cannot prepare you for an explosive snap from calm, status-quo existence to earth-rumbling panic. Words cannot impart the feeling of life suddenly being ripped out from under your feet. Until you've experienced anaphylaxis or witnessed anaphylaxis, the words used to explain and describe the experience are just words.

Feeling the impotence of the words deeply, I attempt each explanation of anaphylaxis with the nagging thought in the back of my mind, "anaphylaxis, now how do I describe this?" Yet try to explain it I must . . . to family members, friends, neighbors, babysitters, school teachers, classmates, parents of classmates, bus drivers, after-school activity directors and so on. Basically every last person who could potentially bring food into my children's lives gets my speech. And then there's the random person I find next to me on a bus somewhere who will never come into contact with my children. Sometimes he gets my speech too. Why? Maybe for practice. Maybe for lack of conversation. Maybe, like all of us, sometimes I just need to share my struggles in life with a stranger.

It is every mother's job to protect her children from harm and for me that means giving my speech. And so I start, "This may sound strange to you, but I need you to listen and take what I say very seriously. My child is severely allergic to food which contains any amount – no matter how small – of nuts of any kind, AND he's allergic to food which contains any amount – no matter how small – of milk protein . . . that includes all dairy products like milk, cheese, ice cream, butter." "Does that include yogurt?" the listener often interrupts. "Yes, yogurt is made from milk and does contain milk protein." "How about soy milk?" they sometimes keep going. "No, actually soy milk is fine. We're just talking about the milk which comes from a cow."

"Please, I'm not asking you to figure out what to feed my child. I actually am asking you NOT to feed my child anything other than food I provide for him. However, I do need you to know what an anaphylactic reaction looks like and how to respond in case my child accidentally eats something containing milk or nuts." "Oh, ok," the listener draws closer, "what happens?" "Well, in my experience, the reactions have been instantaneous. My child seems to know within seconds of eating food containing nuts or milk that he is in dire trouble. Generally, a look flashes across his face like someone has just unplugged his life support system. He typically starts gasping for air and coughing a little with each attempt to draw breath. He has in the past grabbed or scratched at his throat and indicated he could not swallow well. Sometimes his lips and tongue swell up and he starts to drool. Sometimes he breaks out in hives on his face or body. Here's the bottom line: there will be an undeniable look of fear in his eyes, like the look in the eyes of a drowning child. He will be pleading with you to help him – verbally if he can talk, with his eyes if he cannot. And this is what you'll need to do . . . ."

I stop and reflect on my simplified explanation of this complicated physiological reaction. Did any of that make sense? How many times I must have tried to explain my children's anaphylactic reactions! And yet my explanations somehow always fall flat. My explanation never comes close to describing the nearness of death . . . or capturing the nature of the threat. Just as I once choked on the word "anaphylaxis" itself, I now almost always choke on the description. At least the emotions seeping out of my explanation come close to the true experience.

I've spent eight years growing into the role of Food Allergy Mom, all the while trying to understand the actual nature of the threat. The what-is this, how-is-this, why-is-this, and the what-do-we-do-now nature of the threat. As most parents of children with food allergies will tell you, many answers to these questions simply raise more questions. And thus the problem feeds on itself.

Depending upon the source, somewhere between 7 and 12 million Americans suffer from food allergies with the most common food allergens being milk, eggs, peanuts, tree nuts (almonds, hazelnuts, cashews, walnuts, etc.), fish, shellfish, soy and wheat. Each year food induced anaphylaxis is linked to 30,000 emergency room visits and between 150 and 200 deaths. Food allergies appear to be more common among children than adults. The medical community estimates that six to eight percent of children under the age of two suffer from food allergies with milk, eggs and peanuts accounting for 85 percent, whereas only 1.5 percent of adults are considered to have food allergies. For adults the most troublesome foods are tree nuts, peanuts, shellfish and fish.

Beyond this broad overview of the afflicted population, there are few straight answers from pediatricians to the most burning questions regarding food allergies like . . . how and why do some people develop allergies and others do not? Why do allergic reactions differ in nature and severity from one episode to the next? How can one prevent an allergy from developing in the first place? How can one overcome a food allergy? When a person is said to "have grown out of his allergy" what physiological shift has actually taken place and what can we do to make that shift happen?

To ask these questions is to invite an imperious frown from the food allergy community – the doctors and the non-profit organizations whose livelihoods are built upon the premise that food allergies are managed (with the help of professionals like themselves) not cured. The task at hand, in their minds, is not to question the permanency of allergic conditions but to submit to the awesome responsibility of avoiding the worst case scenario - anaphylaxis. As it turns out, with that one word I had been ushered into a fiercely indoctrinated sisterhood of mothers raising children who literally live one bad food-choice away from a near-death experience. With stakes that high, the question isn't how does one get out of this predicament. It is how does one get through the day without her child becoming one of the 150 to 200 people who perish each year from a food-induced allergic reaction.

So, with nowhere else to turn, I joined the club and attacked my assigned responsibilities like a dutiful schoolgirl. Read the medical literature. Check. Safeguard the living environment. Check. Learn to read food labels and prepare safe food for the children to eat. Check. Check. Place Epipens and Benadryl strategically throughout the house and in the car. Check. Practice using the Epipens on old fruit, and when possible call friends or caretakers over for a demonstration. Check. Check. Watch videos and read books and buy medical alert bracelets for the children. Check. Check. Check. And guess what? Despite it all – all the literature I read, all the checklists I followed, and all the explanations I forced on people – despite it all, anaphylaxis still got to my children.

"But that's the unfortunate nature of food allergies, the unfortunate nature of the struggle," say the medical doctors and experts in the food allergy community as they empathize with your feelings of being doomed to a state vulnerability to circumstances which cannot be controlled 100% of the time. Then they pat you on the back and remind you of what a good job you have done the other 99.99% of the time.

Then somewhere along the way a corner was turned and the nature of the struggle changed, not my children's struggle but mine, the Food Allergy Mother's struggle. Episode by episode by episode and close call by close call by close call, I began to sense the presence of an unidentified newcomer to the caldron of emotions. After each panic had passed, after the tears of helplessness had been wiped away, and after yet another threat had been survived there lingered the outline of a stranger which with time came into full view. Anger.

For years the nature of the struggle had been defined by submission and fear and compliance and meekness all in the name of some abstract, clinical condition which had been proclaimed incurable by the medical establishment. But over time the nature of the struggle became personal. Anaphylaxis became a bully on the playground waiting to terrorize my child. And I became one fed-up mother.

It's been quite some time since I was told to make room for anaphylaxis in my life. And in that time a whole lot of room has been made including room in my schedule and creative thinking for the daily task of keeping my children safe ... and room in my reasoning abilities for blood tests and skin tests and baffling and sometimes contradictory test results ... and room in my ego for the humility it takes to request special treatment for my children ... and above all, room in my heart for the look of horror in my children's eyes when anaphylaxis has them by the throat. With all the room I had made in my life for anaphylaxis, it was not hard to find just one inch more for an alternative explanation of allergies - NAET - especially when that explanation offered a possible solution to the problem not at the surface level but at the core.

Note: There is a lapse in time in Susan's Story between diagnosis and the beginning of NAET treatments for her and her children.

She had been so generous with sharing her memories in her very intimate writing style that I asked about the lapse in history which involved several anaphylactic episodes. She responded that she did not want to revisit that time, that it was too painful.

I heartily concurred. She has done a beautiful service in sharing this story with us. Thanks again, Susan. IWP

I first read about NAET in Dr. Nambudripad's book "Say Goodbye to Illness." It was January 2006 and I was taking my first step toward that year's New Year's Resolution: investigate alternative solutions to food allergies. It was a new year and time for a new approach to an old problem. Natalie and Harris were both in school by then and outside the safety of our home for most of the day.

I remember I would inch out of the school parking lot every day with a lump in my throat and a prayer in my heart. Would they be safe out there in a world of unfiltered food choices and a lack of appreciation among the general population for the dangers of food allergies? Of course I always made sure they were wearing their medical alert bracelets, had their emergency kits close by, and that the teachers and parents were constantly reminded of their condition. But I could not find meaningful and lasting peace in that routine forever and I knew it. I wanted out and so I went looking for an exit. If anyone anywhere could tell me they had found a way out, I wanted to hear about it.

Imagine my surprise to find Dr. Prince, one of the premier NAET practitioners in the country, less than ten miles from our house. To me that was more than a coincidence. I wasted no time making an appointment to meet face to face with someone who could explain how NAET works.

Although I had read the book, I would not say that I understood it that well. It was only after experiencing the treatment myself, receiving a personal explanation and rereading the book several times that I began to appreciate the science behind the process of "eliminating" allergies. NAET is - in the truest and most profound sense - an integrative approach to healing, an approach that is derived from a combination of sciences including anatomy and physiology, neurology, physics, and acupuncture. Therein lies the genius of NAET, however, therein also lies the reason a person might dismiss this technique as "too obscure" to merit any consideration. Science has many camps each surrounded by formidable fortresses protecting its own particular explanation of how the world works. NAET bridges the gap between many of these camps.

I was in no particular camp when I came to NAET; I was an outsider. Remember my C in chemistry? Well, I wasn't that much stronger in any of the other sciences, so I had no particular point of view other than that of human sufferer and mother in need of help for her children. Turns out that was the best point of view for receiving the improvements in health NAET offers.

After meeting with Dr. Prince I realized I could benefit from the treatments myself, so Natalie and I began treatment together. It quickly became a bonding experience as we found we both had to have the exact same allergies eliminated. We laughed and talked about the strange sensations we felt in our bodies after each treatment and we kept each other company during the 25 hour avoidance periods. Sometimes we would lie awake together late at night marveling at the overly charged-up state of mental alertness. It can be hard sometimes to get a good night sleep after treatment, but the second night after treatments has always made up for everything.

Natalie and I started our sessions in March 2006 with treatments for BBF and then for eggs. By May we had completed at least ten and were amazed by some of the changes in health we were experiencing, Natalie's being the most rewarding.

Although she was nearly six years old and the beneficiary of excellent education and tutoring, Natalie had been struggling for over a year with little success to fuse the sounds of individual letters into a single, distinct word. She could not read and no one seemed to know why. Within two month's of NAET treatments, this struggle was over. It just evaporated into thin air as if it had never existed. Natalie picked up her books and started sounding out the words as if she had never done anything otherwise.

As rewarding as it was to see her reading it was possibly even more gratifying to see an end to her lifelong battle with eczema. Natalie had suffered from eczema as a baby so badly we had to put socks on her hands at night to prevent her from scratching herself bloody. To keep her scratching to a minimum during the day, Natalie had taken a daily dose of Zyrtec and had to be covered in Aquaphor – a greasy, Vaseline-like topical cream – for many years. Even to this day she still has scars on her body as a testament to her discomfort during those early years. After several NAET treatments, Natalie's skin healed up beautifully and we threw away her Zyrtec.

I too experienced my own personal rejuvenation in health after just a few months of NAET treatments. Although I had not sought NAET treatments to address any one particular complaint, I did have general health issues common among the broad population of stressed-out mothers in their late thirties and early forties: flagging stamina, poor digestion and circulation, headaches, chronic back pain, itchy, red eyes,

nasal congestion and difficulty sleeping through the
am writing this – a little over two years after my first
NAET treatment – I have to stop and think hard to remember
how lousy I used to feel on a daily basis. I certainly still do
experience moments of stress and fatigue today, but on a daily
basis a level of health has been restored that I never would
have dreamed possible before NAET.

By the summer of 2006, Natalie and I were thrilled with
the progress we had made through NAET and I was eager
to start treatments for Harris, only we had to spend most of
June and July in New York City. Fortunately we found another
fabulous NAET practitioner there: Dr. John Crandall. He knew
Dr. Prince personally and welcomed Natalie, Harris and me
as his patients for the six weeks we were in New York. We
were fortunate to have found Dr. Crandall as quickly as we
did because Natalie did not adjust well to all the pollutants
in the big city. Dr. Crandall's treatments eliminated Natalie's
symptoms and allowed us to enjoy a fun-filled summer in New
York.

Dr. Crandall's treatments also launched Harris's journey
toward eliminating his severe dairy allergy. Harris required
fewer basic treatments than Natalie and I had, therefore he
was able to move along quite quickly with his treatments.
Of the top thirty food items on the treatment chart, Harris
required only ten eliminations. By the time we left New York
and returned to Charlotte, Harris had been cleared all the way
up to amino acids.

Dr. Prince was then able to pick up where Dr. Crandall
left off and address Harris's severe allergy to anything with
milk protein in it. Harris's reactions in the past had ranged
from violent vomiting to hideous swelling of his face, lips and
tongue to difficulty breathing. Needless to say, I was terrified
of any dairy products getting anywhere close to Harris. There
are no words to describe how I felt in the fall of 2006 when
Harris was given his first glass of milk in Dr. Prince's office

and no reaction occurred. I was speechless. The struggle had been so long and emotional, yet the resolution was achieved so effortlessly and unceremoniously and without fanfare. It was as if we had been fiddling with a ring of a thousand keys searching for one to unlock the door of our prison and finally one plain, simple key released the lock and set us free. Milk never harmed Harris again.

We continue to this day to rely on NAET treatments and testing to help us overcome health issues. After approximately 20 treatments for peanuts and peanuts in combination with other allergens, Harris (a Class 6 for peanuts) was able to hold a peanut in his mouth with no reaction (see picture below). By the time we reached that milestone, nothing shocked me anymore with NAET. I have witnessed so many personal mini-miracles over the past two-plus years that I have almost become nonchalant about the results. Natalie continues to make progress with her environmental allergies, recently rid herself of an ugly wart on her finger with NAET and looks forward to getting her own treatment for nuts and peanuts as her immune system strengthens.

The world has become a much less frightening and baffling place now that I am aware of NAET. It is there for anyone who can open themselves to the healing possibilities of the human body. As complicated and confusing as sickness can be, sometimes the greatest hurdle to getting better lies in our ability to accept a simple solution

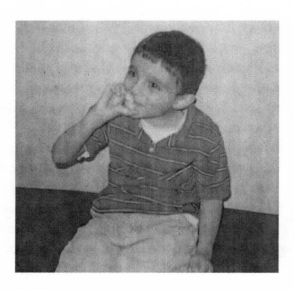

Picture of Harris Patnaik kissing a peanut (not chewing)

Note from another mother Whose sons have Peanut and tree nut allergies

7/0/2008

My boys both have severe peanut and tree nut allergy, which is a contact allergy. I was very nervous about the contact aspect part of the allergy, and did everything I could to best protect them. My son had an allergic reaction when he was not quite two. Shortly after that, I began researching the allergy. When I read about NAET I decided I would try it. I did the treatments for my son/sons and watched my oldest son hold a peanut at the end of his treatments. (Allergy test had him at 6+ on peanuts prior to NAET, I+ when retested several months after completion of NAET.) I have kept up the maintenance part of the treatment, and had them periodically retested.

I believe the treatment has made their systems stronger to the resistance of a potential reaction. After all, I am certain after nine years they have come into contact with it one way or another. I have never, nor would I ever feed peanuts or tree nuts to my children, but I certainly feel good that I did the treatments. I feel like anything you can try to help better safeguard them the better.

T. B. North Carolina

Note: We do not recommend purposeful exposure to peanuts or tree nuts after NAET treatments when the allergy has been severe; however NAET does seem to offer protection against inadvertent exposure. RMP

FOLLOWING ARE SOME RESPONSES FROM OUR PATIENTS. WE HAD ASKED FOR THEIR COMMENTS ABOUT EITHER GOOD OR BAD RESULTS THEY HAD NOTED FROM THEIR NAET TREATMENTS. YOU MAY READ THEM AND DECIDE FOR YOURSELVES HOW VALUABLE THIS TREATMENT HAS BEEN FOR THEM.

Note: These are organized roughly into similar categories since the reader may want to come back for review of situations that more closely apply to themselves.

SECTION A. ARTHRITIS & ALLERGIES IN ANOTHER FAMILY MEMBER

Arthritis; allergies to newspaper, grass, etc.

July 5, 2008
Dear Dr. Bob

During Christmas 1998, my sister told me about NAET. I was being treated by a medical doctor for arthritis with prescription meds and physical therapy. In addition, I was taking calcium/magnesium supplements. My condition was getting worse and worse. I no longer enjoyed dentistry due to the stress of practice and the soreness from the disease. After less than 20 NAET treatments, the symptoms were gone and I could practice without joint pain. We even found that I was severely allergic to the supplements I was taking!!!

While growing up, I started carrying newspapers and mowing grass in our small town. I was found to be highly allergic to both newspapers and grass---BUT NO MORE!!!!! I was so excited that I went to Buena Park and took another practitioner to be trained by Dr. Devi.

During the ensuing years, I have treated many members of my family and referred over one hundred of my patients to the local NAET practitioner. My youngest son was cured of his sleep apnea. One of my assistants had a baby girl who vomited everything she was fed. The doctor wanted to do surgery to place a sphincter on the opening to her stomach to prevent her from throwing up. He even said that the sphincter would come off if she vomited too violently and require another surgery to replace it. After several NAET treatments for food allergies, the baby stopped vomiting completely---NO SURGERY---NO SPHINCTER!!!!

One of my daughters was bitten by a brown recluse spider---she had complete recovery with no tissue damage after NAET treatment.

One of my patients had suffered from milk allergy all his life---over 45 years. NAET stopped the mouth ulcers he got from milk products.

While visiting Dr. Prince's Friday clinic, I met a man with diabetes---AND one LEG cut off!!! He told me that he had had a sore on the other leg and the doctors had planned to cut it off too----UNTIL the NAET treatments enabled the leg to totally heal.

We have used NAET to treat allergy to anesthetic and epinephrine(adrenaline) on many of my patients. This has made it where the patients' pulse does NOT increase after given anesthetic with epinephrine even though it had increased previously.

I have had 3 patients have panic attacks while having dental treatment and each attack was stopped by closing their gates. Each time, we were able to continue treatment within 5 minutes.

I hope this will be beneficial—AND hope you and your family are doing well!!!! Your help has sure changed our lives-—I now have a new office with my oldest son as the manager and we are doing over twice as much business as ever before with very few physical problems thanks to NAET and YOU!!!!!!!!!!!!!!!!!!!!

Rick Jackson, DMD West Columbia, SC

Note: Dr. Jackson had sold his dental prior to getting NAET treatments about 9 years ago.   He was still in his 40's at that time. As you can see from his letter, he was so impressed with NAET that he went to California to be certified as an NAET practitioner. After he was able to resume another independent dental practice, I thought he no longer gave NAET treatments, but, his letter indicates that he still uses NAET when applicable to his dental practice.

Next is a letter from his niece, whom he treated several years ago. RMP

Multiple food allergies; dermatitis, headaches, upset stomaches, and "spacey thughts:

4/28/2008

I spent my childhood sick with sinus problems and "lived on Ampicillin" for the first 18 months of my life due to recurring ear infections. I was unaware of any other issues except for feeling dizzy after eating certain foods, among them: fish, shellfish, pork, honey, artificial sweeteners, and many others. However, even though I did not know why I felt sick after eating sometimes, I didn't question it and just considered it a part of life.

At age 14, I developed atopic dermatitis. It manifested itself on my legs and inner elbows in a red, flaky rash which "weeped" when scratched. And I did scratch it in my sleep. I would wake with scabs and blood under my nails. Mom tried everything for me, including moisturizers, lotions, and hydrocortisone cream. Nothing worked. Finally, when my legs looked so ulcerated that I was embarrassed to wear anything but long pants, my mother took me to an allergist. He prescribed a steroid cream and set me up with testing. I showed allergic to everything on the test except for salmon and sycamore trees. The allergist said the eczema could be related to a food allergy. Nothing else was done for me. When I was tested again 10 years ago, I had the same allergies, only they were worse. The test for dust mite allergy was literally off the chart. I was put on allergy shots but they ended up just making me sicker.

I spent my college years having headaches, sinus infections, rashes, upset stomach and "spacey" thoughts. I was frustrated by the problems I had but I saw no way to stop them. Years later, my aunt began NAET therapy. She sang its praises and my uncle was skeptical but curious. After being treated himself, my uncle realized NAET was for real. He got certified in NAET and began treating our family. After I was tested at Dr. Prince's office in Charlotte, my uncle began treating me. The skin rashes disappeared after I was treated for corn. The headaches and sores in my mouth related to an itchy palate disappeared after I was treated for dust and dust mites. I used to experience nausea, dizziness and headaches if I had even half a cup of coffee. Alter being treated for coffee, caffeine and chocolate, I could drink any beverage I chose, including coffee. After I was treated for sweeteners, I could enjoy things I'd been unable to enjoy before. I no longer had to say "no thank you" at birthday parties when it was time for cake and ice cream.

Another problem I had was feeling dizzy, nauseated and lightheaded after dental appointments. I thought it was the fluoride or the flavoring in it that was making me feel so sick. I could never wear earrings as a teen but was finally able to get my ears pierced after being treated for minerals (a good thing, since before that, I was allergic to my wedding band!

I think the biggest change, though, was when I was treated for fish, shellfish, and iodine. I found out that I would have a reaction to any food cooked with shrimp, such as fried chicken, since it was fried in the same grease. After the first treatment for fish and shellfish, I went to Red Lobster with my coworkers, who knew of my allergy. I got a variety plate and ate it all with no stomach trouble at all. The strangest "treatment" I had done was for a house into which I was moving. I was viewing the house for rent and came down with a horrible headache and dizziness. I knew there was something in the house to which I was allergic, but not specifically. I set wet paper towels in several rooms and got treated with them before my move. I didn't react to the house at all after that!

After I had surgery last year I went for allergy testing and the test results were nothing short of miraculous: I had a slight reaction to dust mites. My body reacted to NOTHING ELSE. (Considering how horrible my dust mite allergy was before

NAET, this really is something.) Even things for which I was not treated didn't cause a reaction. My body has obviously healed itself, and I'm very pleased with the results! (PS - I haven't had even one sinus infection since my dust mite allergy treatment!

Katie Rodriguez Hartsville, SC

SECTION B. ASTHMA

Asthma and son with stomach aches and swollen extremities

7/01/2008

My suffering from attacks of asthma every fall and a child who could hardly eat because of stomach aches, caused a friend to suggest that we look into the NAET treatment. I tossed the information to the side due to it being, I thought, just another gimmick. I went four more years suffering and so did my son. Then an emergency sent my son to the doctor with swelling feet and hands. The diagnoses was allergic reaction to red food dye. We were told he had to stop eating anything with red food dye. My mind was changed and I talked to my friend and listened to her results and we made an appointment. Since our treatments, my son can eat without stomach aches or fear of swelling and my asthma is gone. I feel the NAET treatment has saved our lives and we continue to use it and recommend it.

R. Freeman

Asthma with allergies to cats, grass and pollen

Dear Dr. Prince,

One of the most effective and life changing NAET treatments that I received involved an allergy to cats. The allergy was so severe that if I entered a home with a cat in it or if I was touched by a person who had held a cat I would develop severe rashes in the neck area and asthma. The NAET treatment was so effective for the cat allergy that through a series of events I ended up with a kitten as my pet. He became the best pet I have ever had and it was great to pet him and keep him inside the house without having to deal with asthma or horrible rashes. Another area where NAET improved my life had to do with grass and pollen allergens. I used to have to take a lot of antihistamines to be able to mow the lawn or to do outside activities certain times of the year. I seldom take any antihistamines now, sometimes not even one a year.

Thank you for being the blessing that you are and have been to so many people.

A.H. NC.

SECTION C: AUTISM

December 11, 2005

To Whom It May Concern:
I am writing this letter to praise the efforts of Dr. Robert Prince and his staff at NAET of Carolina. Our son was diagnosed with autism in November of 2001. As you can

imagine, this was devastating news to our family. However, we were glad to finally know what was going on with him. He wasn't eating a variety of foods. His verbal skills were extremely limited. He made very little eye contact, and he did quite a bit of stimming. When we heard of Nambudripad's Allergy Elimination Technique, we researched the Internet for a practitioner that would provide the service. We chose Dr. Prince and his staff because of their level of education in the use of the allergy elimination technique.

We set up an appointment as soon as possible, and Dr. Prince evaluated our son to see how to help him. He recommended that we begin by going through a list of 25 allergens for children with autism spectrum disorder at the time. Once our son began receiving treatments, we were amazed at the improvements that we started to see. We would drive from Raleigh to Charlotte (2 ½ hours) each weekend to see Dr. Prince. That is how impressed we were and still are now. Our son received treatment for the first 25 allergens and more. He is now eating a variety of foods. His verbal skills have improved. He makes better eye contact, and he no longer stims. This year our son is in a regular education kindergarten classroom, and we still go to see Dr. Prince. I highly recommend his services. It changed our lives.

Sincerely,

Rayshawn D. Lockhart   Raleigh, NC

June 2008

Our son was diagnosed with autism at 3 1/2 years old. He began speech & occupational therapy and made some *improvements. He started the NAET treatments with Dr. Prince in March of 2005 [at age 7]. He continued for approximately 18 months. His behavior improved; as did his speech. He began engaging in conversation with people more and speaking in sentences. He seemed to be more "in tune" with his surroundings. We feel Dr. Prince & his staff have a genuine concern for helping our son.*

C.C. & S.C., Charlotte, NC

SECTION D: ECZEMA & SKIN CONDITIONS

Eczema with water & food allergies
June 21, 2008

Dr. Prince,

My daughter, Gabriella, seemed to be allergic to everything she ate or even got close to. As soon as we started feeding her baby food we noticed terrible rashes all over her body. She clawed at her skin sometimes until it bled. We tried for months to determine what she was eating that made her react this way. As soon as we thought we had figured it out, the skin reactions would start again. As an Upper Cervical Chiropractor I had helped thousands of people eliminate allergies and allergic reactions to all kinds of things. But, I could not get my daughter to hold an adjustment for more than a couple of days, she was not getting any better and I was about to lose hope. Until one day a patient of mine shared with me her remarkable experience from seeing Dr. Prince at the NAET clinic in Charlotte, NC.

I made an appointment to see Dr. Prince. At first, like most people I'm sure, I was very skeptical. But, everything that Dr. Prince said made sense to me and we were willing to give it a try. After going through just a few of the basic treatments we started to see a change in Gabriella's skin. She started sleeping better and was much less irritable. In no time Gabriella could eat anything she wanted with no reaction at all. But, there was still a problem. - every time she took a bath she cried out in pain and itched uncontrollably. Getting her in the tub was a nightmare. Getting her to get her head wet or wash her hair was out of the question. We had to use a spray-in hair wash just to try to clean her hair. I bought a very expensive whole-house water filtration system with ultraviolet lights trying to purify the water hoping that would help. No change! I told Dr. Prince about this at one of our visits. He asked that I bring in a small glass bottle of our water on the next visit. He treated her using that water, told us to wait 25 hours before we exposed her to our water again. I was amazed. NO REACTION to the water at all. After getting over her fear of the water she began bathing, washing her hair and playing in the tub until we drug her out. I would have never imagined she could have been allergic to our own, purified water. But, it was true. Dr. Prince desensitized her to it and she has loved the water ever since.

By the way, Gabriella went from holding her Upper Cervical adjustment one to two days to holding it for months at a time. I believe that the allergic reaction she was having to the food she ate and the water stressed her system out so much that she couldn't hold her adjustment. As a result, I have referred several of my patients to Dr. Prince when I noticed they were having a hard time holding their adjustment.

I would like to thank Dr. Prince and his wonderful staff for helping our daughter become the beautiful, happy, healthy little girl that was once so miserable. NAET really did miracles for Gabriella's allergies. I know that NAET has also been very successful helping with Autism, ADD/ADHD, Asthma and many other conditions (that's just the A's). I encourage everyone to go through the NAET program if you or your children are not as healthy as you think you should be. It works!

Dr. Ray Drury

Eczema (daughter) – food & environmental allergies

May 2008

Since my daughter was 4 months old she was plagued with very severe eczema. It started right after I weaned her from breast feeding. For over 8 months afterwards she really suffered. When she was 1 year old she got tested for allergies and of the 40 or so things they tested her for she was very allergic to about 25 of them and moderately allergic to about 10 of them which just left me with practically nothing to feed her. Even with all the control we could exercise she still had severe eczema. To the extent that if I broke open an egg in her vicinity she would start itching or if she would even hold a pecan she would swell up. Antihistamines were her everyday answers to just being a little comfortable. There were days when we changed her clothes more than twice a day since she would scratch herself and bleed. By the time she was 2 we were really at our wits end as to what we should do for her. That was when we moved to Charlotte. Well here she started showing signs of severe environmental allergies also. If we went out and the neighbor was mowing his lawn she would be itchy!. The Allergist started her on Allergy shots. Around this time she could eat about 4 or 5 things only and her eczema was in some control. She would eat Rice, some legumes, potatoes and milk and we would see a little breakout. I was practically every day at the Health Food store looking for Wheat and Gluten free stuff to feed her. What always broke my heart was that she would look at it with such longing when we or her older brother ate anything and would ask for that and we had to explain that it was not good for her. Around the same time I met somebody who told me about NAET. I did some looking up on the Internet and found we had a physician right here. I think that is when my daughter's luck literally changed. We met up with Dr. Prince and he held up a lot of hope that she would be fine. The treatment sounded weird but I was willing to try anything. I refused to let too much logic or lack of an open mind come in the way of helping my daughter (if this could). I noticed a remarkable change in her after a few treatments itself. The Self Treatment method was a blessing it helped me a lot. Every time after a treatment we could try something new for her to eat. The best for us was when she got over her wheat allergy. She would not stop eating bread that day !!! It has been a year and a half now since she has been taking treatment. I can feed her everything she could not have before, and I don't have to carry around stuff for her to have! She still gets mild outbreak of allergies but that is related to the clothes she wears or Pull-Ups. But with self- treatment I have noticed that the breakout heals pretty quickly if I have treated her for the allergen. She happily goes to preschool and eats everything provided there. I thank NAET everyday for being there and for Dr. Devi for bringing this process and working towards helping people with it and Dr. Prince (Ms. Leslie and Ms. Selena his staff) for faithfully following the process and ensuring success.

I would like to add that seeing the results of my daughter a few of my friends have started the treatment because SEEING IS BELIEVING. Also my son and I myself have been doing NAET for our allergies and I am working towards getting rid of my seasonal allergies which are considerably less than last year. I would have no problem sharing my daughter's experience with other parents. I can be contacted via my email at: deepikama@yahoo.com

Thank You again NAET, Dr. Devi, Dr. Prince, Ms. Leslie and Ms. Selena.

Hives, joint pain anaphylactic shock, panic, dental pain

June 2008

In 1997, I began to have occasional hives. They were worrisome but not overly troubling. I had just moved into a new house and given up an 18 year career in the custom drapery business where I handled chemically treated fabrics five days a week.

As my hives increased, a general practitioner referred me to an allergist. The diagnosis was chronic hives, which caused me to test positive for everything. The only treatment was antihistamine taken daily to control the itching. After five years of daily use of antihistamine and the knowledge my condition was worsening,

I had an episode of anaphylactic shock and was rushed to the hospital. After this experience, I began having panic attacks.

I became home bound, unable to eat in restaurants or shop for clothing or food. Even closeting myself in a controlled environment did not stop my reactions. It only lessened the severity of them.

In 2002, I had given up the hope of finding help. I just wanted to die and end the misery. Then a patient of Dr. Prince

told me about NAET treatments. I did not understand how the treatments worked but in desperation I was willing to try. When tested at NAET, I was found to be allergic to every allergen they tried. My body had decided everything was the enemy.

Slowly NAET treatments began to rebuild my health. It has been five years since I was introduced to NAET treatments. During this time, my hives have gone away and other health problems I considered minor under the circumstances have been healed. They include joint pain, ringing ears, sinus problems, burning feet, constipation, depression, acid stomach and chronic bronchial infections.

My last complaint was a dental crown that was sensitive from the beginning, but recently became very painful when hot or cold touched it. After Vitamin D 1,25 treatments, my tooth is doing great. Also, my husband had hip pain and was found to be allergic to leather. His hands were easily bruised and became better after treatment for artificial sweetener. When my grandchildren came along NAET treatments were used for rashes, stuffy sinuses and formula allergies with great success.

Words can never express my gratitude to Dr. Robert Prince, his wife Iris and his wonderful staff for their dedication to patient care and their willingness to explore alternative medicine, If I had known about NAET treatments when my hives began, the allergen would have been identified and treated quickly saving years of suffering. Better late then never!

J. Edwards   Marshville, NC
Hives - daughter
March 1, 2008

When Dr. Prince asked me to write a little something about my experience with NAET, I was more than happy to oblige. NAET has been a great tool for health in my life. I found out about it through a friend of my husbands in the fall of 2000. I immediately made an appointment. I have been a faithful believer in NAET since my first treatment. It has made a "big" difference in the way I view everything regarding energy and has helped me tremendously throughout the years.

I am still amazed at the power of the body every time I go in for a treatment. The results aren't always immediate and sometimes require patience; other times the results are within minutes and it is very exciting.

The first couple of years, I went through the majority of the treatments. Now I go or self treat when I find something that is causing me problems. Some of my most recent visits I have taken my 2 ½ year old daughter. She doesn't seem to have a lot of allergies but when she has one, it is obvious. The most recent one was when she developed really bad hives all over her arms, legs, and face. She had reacted to a combination of herbal products we were giving her for a bad cold. We treated her for them at home and couldn't figure out why they weren't going away. When I took her into the NAET office, through kinesiology, they figured out the piece of the puzzle and treated her for it. It was obvious after the treatment that that was the missing key. The hives had come upon her a few weeks prior to that visit and after that final treatment they were totally gone a couple days later.

I really believe in the power of NAET. If I told you about all of the positive experiences I have had with NAET. I could write my own book. NAET is a "great tool for health". As a Christian, I think it is a gift from God. When used in combination with other forms of holistic treatment and living, it is even more powerful. I know it will be a part of my health regimen for the rest of my life.

Dr. Prince and his staff have been a true blessing to me and my family!

Blessings in health,

Hope Conner Charlotte, NC

Psoriasis

May 5, 2008

Dear Dr. Prince:

After my wife and I completed the basic protocol of NAET treatments, we were treated for a variety of allergies with great success. One outstanding example was my NAET treatment for psoriasis located on my right knee. At first, I went to my dermatologist for possible treatment. He wrote for me a prescription for some very strong cortisone. I decided to try NAET treatments instead of the cortisone. After one or two NAET treatments, my psoriasis disappeared and has not returned for approximately ten years. When my dermatologist saw that the psoriasis was healed without cortisone, his comment was that the NAET treatments were fine with him, because this alternative treatment was successful. Thanks to NAET and Dr. Prince.

Sincerely,

Wayne E. Sterling, Ph.D. Statesville, NC

Note: Most cases of psoriasis do not clear as quickly as did Dr Sterling's. He had been treated for basic allergens and then required only two treatments for the psoriasis vial while touching his fingers to the skin lesions. RMP

SECTION E. ENVIRONMENTAL ALLERGIES

Environmentals; corn tassels & grass

April 29, 2008

Dear Dr. Prince,

In response to your request for comments on NAET treatments I have received at your office, I offer the following:

I first knew I had allergies when my eyes swelled shut the first day of detasseling season in Iowa when I was 16 years old. (Detasseling involves walking through a corn field to pull the pollen-producing tassels out of the top of certain rows of the crop so that only the pollen from another variety of corn that is also planted there will pollinate the corn.) I remember going to a doctor then and getting an inhaler, eye drops, nose drops and pills, the combination of which was effective enough to help me finish working that season and for a couple of seasons after that. Some years later, after I moved to the west coast, I discovered that I was allergic to other kinds of plants, such as scotch broom. I bought eye drops and over-the-counter medicines and got along as best I could in the spring and fall. When I moved to Colorado in the early '90s, I found that I rarely had allergic reactions to anything, and soon forgot about allergies.

I moved to Charlotte from Colorado in 2005, and I noticed that I had much more severe allergic reactions here to pollen. Also, molds have turned out to be a big problem for me here. I had been urged by a good friend of mine who had gotten good relief of her many serious allergies from the treatments to try NAET. She had explained the process to me, and even demonstrated it to me at home. I had also seen how it had helped her. Still, I was a little skeptical. Frankly, it did not make any sense to me how it could work. I also felt that my allergies were really not that bad, since I had been able to function for years with them. I considered them to be more of an inconvenience than anything. Still, my much worse symptoms in Charlotte finally drove me to try NAET in early 2006.

Having now gone through the course of the initial treatments and treatments for more of the specific allergens, I have gotten excellent relief. I have had to be treated for grasses several times (corn is a kind of grass, as you know), but other things I have been treated for have not again caused me any further trouble. The treatments have been so effective that I have been able to regularly mow four acres of the grounds at my church, even though much of that land is filled with grass, ragweed and other plants that formerly would cause me to sneeze and wheeze and itch. There are several other things I have found I am allergic to, and I have gotten relief from those as well. I believe that I am less irritable and more patient with others now, too.

I still do not understand exactly why or how NAET works, but I can say that it does work, and that is good enough for me. Thank you and your staff for all the help and kindness you have shown me over the past year and a half.

Jay Huldeen Charlotte, NC

Chronic sinus congestion

April 2008

I had mild to moderate allergies living in Michigan. After moving to North Carolina in 1997, I started having severe allergies every spring and fall. I was miserable. My sinuses were always congested. I started with OTC allergy medicine, then to my Primary Care Physician and got a prescription for allergy medicine and then to an allergist and got shots for over a year - never feeling better. I gave up on the treatment and just took Benadryl every day before bed. This went on for a couple of years and helped me from having problem get severe, but I would still get sinus headaches periodically and needed antibiotics if the congestion lasted too long.

I have family that used the NAET treatment, as I have, with success and I am pleasantly surprised to say I don't even notice any congestion since my NAET treatments several years ago. In fact my husband who I used to envy gets more congestion than I ever do. I could write more.

Thank you!
Roberta Anderson, Mooresville, NC

Environmental & emotional issues

July 10, 2008

NAET is an important part of my health care. Our daughter, an NAET practitioner, began treating me about 10 years ago, starting with the NAET basic protocol.

In my late teens, I tested allergic to house dust, feathers, etc., and for years, I received desensitizing allergy injections every two weeks, but this treated the symptoms, not the basic cause.

I have received help from many NAET treatments, but three stand out:

Almost 30 years after I had mononucleosis, I was treated for it by NAET and my energy improved remarkably.

For years, I suffered recurring attacks of acute cystitis and was prescribed antibiotics to be taken 14 days on, seven days off for an extended time. Now, NAET controls the problem.

In June 2002. Dr. Devi's dear sister Mala treated me on the emotional level for grief over my grandmother's death 20 years earlier. I had no idea my body was carrying that stored grief. The relief was truly wonderful.

I am a healthy 74 year old female. I take no prescription or over-the-counter drugs and I lead an active, fulfilling life.

FRANCES L REYNOLDS MONROE, NC

SECTION F: EMOTIONS

Depression, tiredness, fear of eating out and insomnia

June 24, 2008
Hi Dr. Prince

My daughter had been ill for over 10 years. We had tried all medically "accepted" diagnoses and treatments with no results. Even after many years, many hours, and much money, we still had no answer as to her issues. And issues she had! She was depressed, tired, nausea and list goes on. This all started around age 10 and just never improved.

One day a friend of mine mentioned about NAET and this "Dr. Prince". It all sounded pretty weird to me, after all, who can get rid of allergies without any medication or shots? And allergies make you sneeze, nothing else. But by this point, we were willing to try anything! So we called and made the appointment. After our initial appointment with Dr. Prince, he made it clear that the 1st 10 treatments had to be completed before moving on to the issues at hand. I was skeptical but thought we had nothing to lose. So after a few of the initial *treatments, we started noticing some significant changes. She was happier, had more energy and just felt better.*

When she started seeing Dr. Prince, she was on Paxil to try to help her till we could find the problems. Within 6 months she HAD to come off Paxil. Her body did not need it and she could tell. She could tell she was getting better. She had several major changes that really impressed us.

You see, she had stopped eating out at restaurants and all fast food places for many years. She had some sort of fear of getting sick from meat, especially chicken. So if she had to buy something, it would be French fries, but nothing significant. One time, a few days after going for her NAET treatment, she called home. She said, you will never guess what I am doing? My husband and I asked what? She said eating chicken out!

I could not even hold back the tears. I know this doesn't seem like much, but it was amazing!! Years of fear controlling her life had just vanished. And it is still gone! And that is just one thing. Another major milestone was changing her sleeping. She could never sleep! So **after a dopamine treatment, she would sleep all night soundly.** What a difference that makes when you can actually rest! Depression started disappearing, memory problems and the list goes on. The experiences we have had from NAET would fill volumes! The whole family started treatments and have all gone through the initial 10. We all go occasionally now, but no need to go very often. We no longer spend money at doctors with fancy blood test and other stuff. No one is on any medication. And everyone sleeps soundly. We would not be at this point if it was not for Dr. Prince (both of them!).

Words cannot express our gratitude. But we can try, THANK YOU AGAIN!!!

M.R. and family

SECTION G: FATIGUE

Chronic Fatigue Syndrome with food and environmental allergies

June 30, 2008

I'd been disabled by chronic fatigue syndrome for 15 years, with a host of food allergies and environmental sensitivities piled on. A holistic doctor referred me to Dr. Prince for the food allergies. It sounded wacky to me and I approached it with skepticism.

Immediately after my first treatment I felt ill, and spent the 24 hours in bed. How could something so non-invasive affect me so profoundly? I concluded something was going on, and maybe it was good. After about six treatments, a few of my symptoms lessened. I was mystified, but I kept going.

I'd had the best care that western medicine could offer for someone with CFS, but it wasn't enough. The NAET treatments helped me regain some of my life.

KS Charlotte, NC

Fatigue, headaches and hormonal problems

July 2, 2008

I started NAET treatments approximately 3 months ago for chronic, daily headaches and fatigue. I was also having issues with hot flashes, night sweats and mood swings. I had been under the care of my gynecologist for the past 4 years for the above symptoms. The symptoms started after the birth of my only child. I did suffer severe post partum depression for the first year after having my child. My gynecologist had *performed a lot of blood tests, had changed by birth control pill several times, started me on Lexapro and Wellbutrin for a period of time, referred me to a reproductive endocrinologist and performed a hysterostomy. All of the above failed to bring me any relief.*

I did have an IUD put in about 6 weeks before I started the NAET treatment as a last attempt to help my symptoms and was having some difficulty adapting, but once I started the NAET treatments I felt a remarkable improvement in my energy and my headaches began to subside within 2 treatments. I now have had 9 or 10 treatments and my energy level is what it was before I had my child. I am headache free 95% of the time and I feel great. I do notice that the 25 hour period after a treatment I often feel tired and have a headache but I attribute this to my body clearing the substance I was being treated for. The fatigue and headache are nothing more than what I was having a problem with before I started.

My mother had NAET treatments 6 years ago and I have always been open to the idea of alternative and complementary medicine but just got stuck in the traditional medical treatment path since I practice traditional medicine. I also felt a strong rapport with my gynecologist and felt comfortable with his care. I had almost accepted a life of fatigue and headaches, thinking there was no other way. Something made me try NAET. I am not sure what, but I was open to it and it has worked. I have since returned to my gynecologist and have shared my good news and he was happy for me but he was skeptical about the NAET treatments.

Kristin Richline-Elledge, Charlotte, NC

SECTION H. FOOD ALLERGIES

Food (especially milk) & Environmentals

April 2008

When I began NAET treatments in 2001, I was in what I call a hyper-sensitive state in which I was reacting to nearly everything I ate, breathed and came into contact with.

When I first saw Dr. Prince, I was even unable to use toothpaste, shampoos and other similar products without reacting to them. My attempts at addressing these issues were getting increasingly frustrating as I reacted to everything that was prescribed to me to alleviate my symptoms, both by traditional doctors and alternative health care professionals.

I began treatments, driving two hours each way from Blowing Rock to Charlotte twice a week while I was being treated for the Basic 10, I never questioned the length of the trip as I began to see immediate results. After then, I would come once a week until so many of my allergies were eliminated that I gradually decreased the frequency of my trips. I have not been down to the clinic for about two years now and have regained the strength and vitality that was missing from my life for so many years. Of great benefit was the self-training course that Dr. Prince and his wife offer to those patients who have completed the Basic 10, enabling my husband (also an NAET patient) and me to test and treat ourselves.

I have eliminated all of my allergies through NAET except for the milk protein, a condition that has been in my family for generations. Through the ability to self test, however, I am able to eat comfortably in restaurants or while traveling as we can "check" anything that might contain dairy with a simple muscle test. Needless to say, I feel as if my life has been given *back to me and I now have the freedom to travel and eat out in restaurants without worry.*

Dr. Prince and his staff were always kind and helpful and always took as much time as I needed, especially in those first few weeks. During my visits to the clinic, I especially enjoyed the room where everyone sits for 15 minutes after having been treated before going home. It was so interesting to share stories with the other patients and extremely encouraging to know how so many people, many with very serious medical conditions, were being helped by this simple procedure.

I owe a great deal of thanks to Dr. Prince and his staff who gave me the tools to get my life back on track. I know many others share in my gratitude to him and everyone at the clinic. My whole family has benefited from NAET, even our dogs!

Nancy Brittelle

Blowing Rock, NC

Multiple food allergies

May 8, 2008

Doctor Prince,

My career is in the food service industry and I was quite often in the position of having to sample food products. It is very difficult to function publicly in food position when you can't eat most of the products.

A letter that I had written to a doctor in California   before I met you explained how my food allergies were intensifying. It listed all of the types of food that I could no longer eat, dairy, beef, pork, many processed foods, MSG, wheat, tomatoes, many fresh vegetables, tea and certainly anything with nitrates in it which gave me intense personal discomfort. The letter was dated early 2003, and I read it after my NAET treatment.

I had been recommended to a food allergy specialist in NY, and he did help me temporarily. I went to him twice per month at a cost of $250.00 per half-hour visit. This doctor identified all of the foods that I had grown allergic to (many of which I had eaten my entire life). After approximately a year, I was feeling stronger, and I had lost an undesirable amount of weight. Many people thought that I had cancer from my appearance. My diet was primarily chicken and rice.

After moving to Charlotte, I had a very good understanding of the few items available on most restaurant menus that I could order. I typically brought spelt bread to restaurants to have served with my meals.

Out of pure desperation, I was in a book store and figured that I would check out new releases for potential cures to my problem. I saw the NAET book and began to read about people who had similar problems that I was experiencing. With a little more research on the Internet, I located your office in Charlotte.

Your office team was wonderful! From the initial phone conversations to office appointments, they were friendly, knowledgeable and supportive. It was a real sense of caring and family.

I must admit, that my first impression of the treatment was that it sounded ridiculous, and I was actually embarrassed to be sitting there "having my gates closed" (I am certain that I am using the incorrect terminology). After the first simple treatments of a few taps on the back, I went home and fell asleep for 12 solid hours. Something affected me, and I was not certain what. Out of desperation, I continued NAET and began to see actual results. Blind faith lead me to actually try and eat food that I would get violently ill over just a few days before. I did try the foods, and was capable of digesting it without ill effect. As

I gained confidence in the treatment, and completed the first 10 groups of food, I began to request products to be treated for based on what I missed the most. At one point, I recall calculating that I had 3 appointments before my vacation, and I wanted to enjoy pizza, beer and ice cream on the trip. Bringing in these items to get treated for also seemed silly, but when my friends (who I saw annually on vacation) witnessed me eating these foods, they were believers.

I did experience some small set-backs on products initially, but was retreated, and the fix has lasted over 5 years. I anticipate that they will be permanent.

My quality of life has increased tremendously! I still have some reservations in the back of my mind that remind me of the problems that I associated with certain foods, such as those containing nitrates and I often hesitate to eat them. Additionally, I should mention that before the treatment when I would get sick on certain ingredients, I was not aware that the ingredients were in the food when I ate it. Only after getting sick did I go back to check the food ingredients to discover what caused the problem. For me, I believe that my problems were physical.

Since my treatment, I have referred many friends and family to NAET. From Charlotte to California, to Connecticut. I have to brace them on how simple the treatment is, and have received many positive responses from them. Countless conversations in the waiting room with other patients validated that what I was experiencing was not unique at all.

The most effective treatment ended up being the least costly. While I certainly did go to hospitals for testing, I can equate my entire cost of NAET treatment to be less than I major test in a hospital. Additionally, I always felt that you and your team were genuinely interested in helping people and enjoyed seeing the positive results that you achieved as much as the patients.

The NAET treatments solved my problems, and also had direct and indirect benefit to my family.
Thank you!
D.M. – Charlotte, NC

Multiple food allergies Son with fatigue; daughter borderline ADD

April 2008

Dear Dr. Prince,

My first visit was in 1999. A friend at work told me about NAET, who heard of it from another friend. I had severe food allergies at the time to the point where I could only eat unseasoned meat, plain rice and some vegetables. I also could not eat anything that contained wheat, food-coloring seasonings. Within minutes of eating, I would suddenly begin to feel like I had the flu. Sometimes I actually ran a low-grade fever. My face would become pale with flushed cheeks. A rash would appear on my neck and my ears would turn bright red. One of the doctors observed this happening as I started to chew gum. I could see the surprised expression on his face as he observed how quickly my symptoms appeared. The two answers to my problems I finally received from Chapel Hill were: 1) Do not eat the food that bothers you. 2) Look for an alternative.

There was nothing that Western Medicine could do for me. It was perfect timing when my friend at work told me about NAET. Her comment was, "What do you have to lose?" Needless to say I decided to make the first appointment.

Dr. Prince explained the process and he treated me for egg allergies, which was the first part of the basic treatment. All I had to do was avoid foods that contained eggs for twenty-five hours. This was the easy part, because all I could eat *was meat and rice. However, several hours later, I began to feel nauseated, dizzy, feverish and fatigued. I lay down and the room felt like it was spinning. I thought to myself, if this is what all the treatments feel like, I'm not sure I can do this. The following day the uncomfortable symptoms subsided. I actually began to feel better. Then I was treated for B-Complex. I was so pleased that I didn't have the same reaction as with the eggs. The most amazing thing is that after being treated for the eggs and B-Complex, I could eat pasta and bread. I was so excited! I continued through the basics and was able to eat again.*

Just recently, I made an appointment for my son, who is 18 years old. He has been seen by a kidney specialist and a gastroenterologist who were unable to find out what was causing the sickness. He was so dehydrated that he almost lost all kidney function. After being in the hospital for nearly a week, which involved undergoing many tests and x-rays, no answers could be found. He continued seeing the same gastroenterologist, but his condition continued to worsen the last several months. He got to the point where he was nauseous and fatigued all day long and had completely lost the desire to eat. I suddenly thought of NAET again and made him an appointment. When Selena worked with him she hypothesized that his symptoms may be stemming from something he smelled at the time. She asked him specifically if he had used a new hair gel or deodorant recently. He had been using, and still was using two products for over one year that he had begun using three months prior to the noticeable beginning of the sickness. Selena gave us instructions on what to do at home, as well as information on the treatments that she would give him in the office. After two treatments, his energy was noticeably better and the nausea began to subside. After the third treatment, he has even less nauseated and had even more energy. It is incredible! The wonderful part is I can see he feels better, his appetite is back and his energy level has greatly improved.

When I brought my son back his eleven-year-old sister came along. She was having trouble in school because of her short attention span and focusing. A questionnaire given by one of her teachers showed she was borderline ADD. I also mentioned to Selena that she tossed and turned at night, changing positions constantly. I could tell she was not sleeping well at night. Once again, Selena worked with her and came up with a game plan. The first treatment showed significant results. My daughter even noticed it. Now after her third treatment, she can focus better at school, sleeps better and cannot wait until her next appointment.

The sad part is that my husband is extremely skeptical of almost everything. Even though he has seen the changes in me and our children, he does not believe it was the treatment that helped. I try to share this with friends who have children with severe allergies, but they don't believe or want to explore the possibilities. It just sounds too good to be true. Both my son and daughter have seen the benefits of the treatments and want to go to appointments, because they know it does work and it makes them feel better.

I truly believe an individual must have an open mind when considering NAET. It is very different from traditional medicine; however, it is based on the most traditional techniques ever discovered. The techniques worked hundreds of years ago and they still work today. I never regret making the first phone call to the clinic in 1999. NAET has been a blessing for me and for my children.

I especially want to thank Dr. Prince, his wife Iris, Selena and the others at NAET of Carolina who have chosen the path to help others heal by using NAET. I also want to thank Dr. Devi S. Nambudripad, who founded the technique, and her commitment to helping others around the globe.

Many thanks,
C.M., Charlotte, NC

Overwhelming food and other allergies

July 14, 2008

Dear Dr. Prince,

NAET has truly made my life immeasurably better! My family has MANY food allergies. Thankfully, none of them is deadly, but all of them contribute to poor health. I had been tested for allergies by a doctor in Charleston, SC, and had found out that I was reactive to a large number of foods that are "good for you" - almonds, avocado, banana, buckwheat, cantaloupe, celery, grapes, lemon, green peas, pinto beans, spinach, squash, string beans, tomatoes, wheat, milk, and eggs. I was also reactive to beef, chicken, and lamb! Benzene, ethylene glycol, formaldehyde, orris root, saccharine, and sodium metabisulfite (red wine and Vienna Fingers!) were reactive as well. This list does not include the things to which my response was "equivocal". Needless to say, I was quite depressed when I received these results.

It was virtually impossible for me to avoid all of these foods. Plus, my family tends to DEVELOP allergies to any food eaten on a regular basis. Therefore, I would soon be reactive to the foods I <u>was</u> allowed to eat. I decided to participate in an experimental treatment for food allergies known as Enzyme Potentiated Desensitization under the care of Dr. John Wilson. I was unable to tolerate the small amount of allergen injected under the skin as a part of this treatment, so treatment was ended. Dr. Wilson said there was nothing else he could do for me, but he said he had heard of new approach to allergies - NAET - and he gave me your name.

To be honest, I was very skeptical about NAET. My mind began to change when NAET computer testing revealed the same allergies that had been identified in my previous testing through ALCAT testing and through skin testing. Prior to my first testing, I asked you, "Do I have to believe in NAET for it to work?" You responded that while belief might be helpful, it was not necessary. I responded that that was a good thing, since I did not believe in it. I do now!

I have now been treated for <u>many</u> items through NAET by you, Rick Sibley, and most recently, my husband. I am happy to say that it has changed my life! When I was treated for Vitamin C, a wide range of foods became healthful for me. I no longer break out in a rash when I eat tomatoes, and I am able to enjoy broccoli, spinach, citrus fruits, and other Vitamin C-rich foods. There is no need to point out that it has made a great difference to be able to eat cheese and other calcium foods without resulting headaches. Prior to NAET, dinner out in a nice restaurant <u>almost always</u> resulted in an evening of diarrhea. Because my allergies were so numerous, it was impossible to determine which allergy actually caused the problem, but as a result of my NAET treatments, I <u>rarely</u> have diarrhea after a meal.

I have also been treated for my inhalant allergies - trees, weeds, and flowers. My ability to be outdoors has greatly improved.

I have far fewer headaches, few food-related migraines, rare digestive reactions to food, few rashes, and simply feel much better overall due to NAET. While I need a touch-up treatment on a few items - eggs, Vitamin B, and magnesium - most of my allergy treatments have held for years. I will be retreating these soon, and I am confident that the treatments will be successful.

Thank you for all you have done to improve my health and the health of so many.

Sincerely,

K.B. North Carolina

Foods, eczema, asthma, cats

June 23, 2008

I had battled food allergies most of my life and those foods I was aware of, I avoided (eggs, cabbage, oatmeal). One that I was not aware of in the early 1990's caused me serious distress. By the time I figured out that soy was the culprit, my skin was so irritated that I appeared to have 2nd degree burns over most of my body. I went to a dermatologist and was treated with steroids and some UV light therapy. My skin cleared up somewhat, although I always looked like I had a sunburn on my face, I itched constantly and didn't want to be touched. I practiced food avoidance to and read labels constantly to keep my allergies somewhat under control.

In 1998 I was 40 and had developed asthma to the degree that I needed a rescue inhaler daily. My asthma and allergy doctor had determined I had allergies to various pollens and dust mites. I took weekly shots for nearly 2 years in an attempt to build up my tolerance to them.

I was at my second yearly checkup with my asthma and allergy doctor in early 2000 and I really wasn't seeing any improvement. I asked him how long I would need to take the shots and the asthma medication. He informed me this was a permanent situation and this would be my way of life from now on. I was not happy with the answer. I do not like to take medications. I never returned to his office. I was determined to find a cure for my problem, not a treatment for the symptoms.

In March of 2000, I saw a documentary on a cable health channel about a doctor in Denver that was treating food allergies with acupressure and that the treatment was actually a cure!

I researched on the internet and found the closest NAET doctor which was only 45 minutes away. Dr. Prince and the NAET treatments were an answer to prayers.

I started treatments and began to see improvement. I had so many allergies, that the results were more gradual for me. I failed all the basic 10 for most of my organs. But after 3 or 4 months of treatments, the change was considerable and my skin was clearer and my asthma symptoms were nearly gone. It was definitely working and I was experimenting with foods I had been allergic to and testing my reactions to reassure myself the treatment was working.

I returned in the fall of 2000 for a few more treatments and then stopped going since I was so much better. I continued to share my story with friends, family and strangers in person and on the internet as the opportunities presented themselves.

I returned to Dr. Prince in November of 2007 to get some additional treatments. I have cats and knew I was allergic but for some reason never asked to be treated. The cat treatment was an immediate success and my eyes stopped itching and I was able to cuddle my cats to my face. I believe my cats appreciated the change in me.

As a result of my return after 7 years, Dr. Prince was able to check my prior treatments and confirm what I already knew, that the treatments were holding. I still have flare ups for unknown allergens, but they usually subside quickly. I will be returning for additional treatments to determine what foods are still bothering me. Thanks to Dr. Prince and his dedicated and caring staff my quality of life is improved dramatically.

Lelane, South Carolina

Chocolate (also ragweed & mold)

June, 2008
I did not believe it would work until I tried it. I was allergic to chocolate. If
I ate any, within five minutes I would have throat drainage and a stuffy nose. After treatment from Dr. Prince, I can now eat all of the chocolate I desire. I was allergic to ragweed and mold until he cured me of that also. As far as I am concerned this is a miracle.

Yours truly,
Pliney Purser Monroe, NC

Allergies to Shrimp, poison oak On long term allergy shots

June 2008

When I first met Dr. Prince in 2006, the subject of my allergic reaction to shrimp was mentioned in our conversation. This gentleman introduced himself as Dr. Prince of NAET of CAROLiNA. He mentioned he might be able to help me with my allergy problem. At that time, I was highly allergic to shrimp. Being highly allergic, developing a rash from head to toe after eating any amount of shrimp prepared in any fashion. I had developed this allergy suddenly about twenty years ago. I was also taking two shot weekly for other miscellaneous allergies.
I had been told by allergy specialist that there was no cure or treatment for food allergies other than avoid contact with the food substance. Being somewhat surprised by his statement of what was believed to be impossible, I was excited

by any possible opportunity to eat one of my favorite seafoods again.

After talking with Dr Prince, I became thrilled that I might once again enjoy my favorite foods.

Being a firm believer in alternative medicine, making an appointment was a must. Still skeptical at my first visit, we further discussed my allergy problems, and began treatment. When I received my first treatment, I almost chuckled to myself, and asked what have I gotten into. Is this some kind of Voo Doo? It was so simple I could not believe it would do any good. After several routine treatments, the shrimp test was next, and I was cleared to eat shrimp. This was scary, first, I held a shrimp in my hand, no reaction. Next day, put a shrimp in my mouth, no reaction. The following day I swallowed a shrimp and had no adverse reaction.

The next week, I got up enough nerve to order a shrimp cocktail and also ate some fried shrimp. After a few hours I thought I was going to have a reaction, so I took some benadryl, and nothing happened. I mentioned this to Dr Prince, and was retreated for shrimp. Since that day, I have been able to eat all the shrimp I care to; without any adverse reaction.

I have continued NAET treatments for other allergies, including poison oak and all the other allergies that I was taking two shots a week to treat. Now, at age seventy-one, I take no allergy shots and am seldom bothered by any allergy conditions. Wish I would have known about this treatment many years ago.

Many thanks to NAET, Dr. Prince, and his staff.

Roy L. Briggs Mount Holly, NC

SECTION I: MEDICATIONS, ANESTHESIA, ETC.

Medication allergies & hives Also reflux and nasal congestion in son

7/7/2008

Dear Dr. Prince,

Thank you so much for asking us to participate in this book.

NAET treatments are remarkable and were the only way that I was able to get rid of my allergic reactions. My eyes and lips used to swell anytime I took any type of antibiotic or pain killer medicine, my list of medication allergies was endless just to name a few... Penicillin, Amoxicillin, Tetracycline, Ceclor, Naprosyn, Erythromycin, Levaquin, Advil, Tylenol, or any generic brand pain killers. Try fitting that on a Medic Alert bracelet... The medical doctors were just baffled by my list and I was told that it was IMPOSSIBLE to be allergic to all these medications. Out of total desperation and frustration, at the advice of my sister who had success with NAET, I tried this crazy allergy elimination technique that we would tease her about tirelessly. It turns out that I was allergic to a filler product in all of these medications. Although I rarely need to take medicine, I can and have done so safely for the past 7 years. It almost sounds too good to be true. But it is true and it is absolutely amazing. My advice, don't think about it too much, just do what they instruct you to do. I was treated on several items over time and felt SO much better! Another big item I was allergic to was shrimp. My face would break out in hives. I have been able to eat it successfully over the past 7 years too.

Our first son was allergic to his formula and seemed to have reflux type issues. We took him to NAET when he was just a few weeks old. He was treated on formula with a few different combinations and treated on the basic 10 items. Before we completed the Basic 10 treatments, his reflux issues and crying spells disappeared. As he cleared these allergies, he did have a few crying spells and I remember him vomiting a time or two (usually within the first 10 hours of the treatment), but I believe it was just his body's way of clearing this allergic reaction. It is all worth it. He has been a very happy and content child. Now he wakes up happy because he isn't congested and he can breathe again! His mood during the daytime has changed drastically from grouchy to happy again!

Our daughter went to NAET after she had immunizations. We took her on the same day as her well-baby check up and she was showing some sensitivity to the shots. She has been cleared on all of these issues.

We are grateful to you, the NAET staff, the NAET method, and all of the help you have given to our family. Thank you again, Dr. Prince!

E.M. of North Carolina

Surgical sutures, Mononucleosis, antibiotics, And animal treatments

7/11/2008   NAET Miracles

About four (4) years ago I had an emergency appendectomy. The following 6 months I suffered rashes and itching that were driving me crazy.   The rash covered almost 50% of *my body. I went to every doctor and specialist I could think of and was given every cream, drug and anything else on the market. One doctor thought I had herpes!! I was in such bad shape I couldn't sleep, couldn't work and was going crazy. Finally one doctor was musing that maybe I could be allergic to the internal sutures from the surgery. It was the first anyone had connected what I had to the surgery, yet I knew all my problems had started then. At the same time I saw an infomercial about NAET and in desperation phoned Dr. Prince's office. They were so kind and understanding and suggested I ask the hospital for samples of the sutures and bring them in right away with me. Within a week the relief was so great I started feeling like a human again. All I could think of was: "What IS this stuff?" Within a couple of weeks my skin was back to normal.*

From there we went back through the basics. The change in my health was drastic. I'd never thought of myself as having any allergies at all and never had problems with grass or weeds or foods. However, as we progressed, there were many other things I had to be cleared of. Some of the most profound was finding Mononucleosis still in my system some 50 years after I'd been hospitalized with an especially bad case of it as a teenager. I was so over-dosed with antibiotics at the time, that I developed an allergy to penicillin and sulfa and my skin turned yellow. I had developed a severe allergy to the drugs and was told NEVER to take these antibiotics for fear of the consequences. Well, you know I was treated the mono and the drugs, and now have no fear if I ever have to have the drugs. I had also quit smoking some 35 years ago, but smoke was found in my lungs and then cleared. I discovered that some of the odd things that I'd put up with all my life were actually allergies that were manifesting as bleeding hemorrhoids, headaches, bloated stomach, indigestion, acid reflux, etc. As each thing was cleared and eliminated I became more excited. The next step was to ask about arthritis and ruptured disks after I read about other people finding pain relief through NAET.   I had had a serious horse accident some 30 years ago that left my spine pushed over ¼ inch and was riddled with 6 ruptured disks. As I have aged, the arthritis and pain had become unbearable. At one point, a chiropractor refused to work on me any more and said I would be in a wheelchair if I didn't have surgery.   I found a new chiropractor willing to work with me who has the new Nasa machines and Leslie and Selena started pinpointing causes and affects and foundational problems NAET could help with. I am blessed to say that in the last year, I am able to get out of bed with relatively little pain in the morning; and I am able to work out and exercise and do things that I have not for many many years.

I could write about 15 more pages on all the things that I and my family have been treated for and had eliminated from our bodies - – –releasing us to live healthier, happier, stronger lives.

NAET in animlals

We have also been guided by Dr. Prince in how to use the NAET on our golden retrievers that are used for therapy and assistance dog work. We have seen one miracle after another in overcoming health setbacks, vaccine reactions and chemical detox.   Again I have dozens of stories about the dogs, but will relate only a couple of the most profound ones. "Autumn" is one of our more experienced and precious therapy dogs. At age 11 one of her eyes started sinking into her skull. The vets diagnosed 'Horner's Syndrome" and said there was nothing that could be done and that occasionally they resolve on their own in 8 weeks or never get better if there is a brain tumor – which is usually the cause.   We treated "Autumn" that night and her eye was nearly normal the next morning and *completely normal in 2 days!! We have cleared the dogs for parasites, vaccines, hot spots, other allergies, radiation after x-rays and anesthetic after surgeries. We combined NAET with some other natural remedies for an elder dog with Hermangiosarcoma. Any vet will tell you that after spleen surgery for this fast growing and fatal cancer, dogs only survive an average of a couple of months.*

Our "Pearl" lived 6 years beyond her hermangiosarcoma surgery and died at the age of 14.5 of simple old age – not cancer.

There are dozens more miracles from NAET that my family and I have seen and experienced in the last 4 years and we can truly say that this methodology has indeed not only changed our health and our lives, but SAVED our lives!

I have no fear of cancer or health problems or alzheimers or any of the other aging matters, because NAET and Dr. Prince and his wonderful staff have balanced our bodies, equipped us to recognize when it is stressed and taught us what to do about it in the most natural, non-invasive way. There just are no finer nor more humble people than Dr. & Mrs. Prince, Leslie and Selena. NAET of the Carolina's is truly the old fashioned caring, careful and dedicated office that loves their patients and wants to see them well in the quickest most inexpensive way. My thanks to them is not enough because how can you adequately thank people who have given you back your life through their knowledge and use of NAET.

Ann Chase Charlotte, NC 28271
P. O. Box 77108
28271

I am happy to speak with anyone who wishes to contact me.

Medications, smoke, also grandchildren with shellfish allergy, ADHD, etc

March 2008

Members of my family and I have been treated successfully for many allergies. 15 or so years ago I was treated by Beth Owens in Denver, CO (NAET - recommended by my grandchildren's pediatrician – the kids can now eat shellfish) – particularly for cigarette smoke. I no longer have any problems when people are smoking normal cigarettes, and I no longer have sinus infections every few weeks. You have treated me successfully for allergies to many medications that I need for various health problems, but could not use before treatment. I have no problems with any of those now.

You have treated one of my grandsons (ADHD), now 14 – he had an almost sudden change in behavior after treatment.

Gerry Bernard   Charlotte, NC

Anesthesia & friend with shellfish allergy

June 21, 2008

Dear Dr. Prince, I really have to say that I am constantly amazed by the results of the NAET treatments.

However when I first came to see you in February of 2003, I must admit that I was very skeptical of this strange new treatment!

Gradually I came to believe in these treatments, and brought my daughter and grandchildren. Especially to help the *grandchildren, by having them treated for their "shots" before they had to have them, to prevent any side effects.*

I also brought a French friend for treatments to help cure her allergies to shell fish and peanuts. After many weeks of treatments her allergies were gone. We even gave her a shrimp to try in your waiting room with everyone watching !!! It worked. We then gave her a small piece of crab meat at home along with a peanut ....and she was fine.

Just recently, I have not been well myself. For four months I was so weak following surgery, I had trouble putting one foot in front of the other. I was treated for many different allergies over a six week period (including the anesthesia from the surgery !!) and I feel like a new person.

So it is with deep and heartfelt thanks to you, Leslie and Selena, that I feel better now than I have in a long time.

Bless you all,
Sally Rojzman, Hickory, NC

SECTION J. HEART ARRHYTHMIA

July 10, 2008

In February 2008, within a 24 hour period I became very sick- high fever, chest pains, shortness of breath and was very weak.

I went to the emergency room that evening and was diagnosed with the flu and pneumonia. I was hospitalized in ICU due to heart arrythmia which the doctor said was brought about by the infection.

My infection improved, but five days later there was no change in the arrythmia despite the usual drugs to correct it. The doctor discussed using shock to restore normal heart rhythm. I refused this treatment due to lack of positive data regarding long term effect of keeping the heart in rhythm.

Our daughter is an NAET practitioner, but was not with me much because her young daughter was home sick with the flu, also.

Finally, our daughter was able to muscle test me and within 12-15 hours of being treated for my granddaughter's saliva (who also had a high fever and the flu) my heart rhythm returned to normal during the night.

The smiling nurse who watched the heart patterns on the monitor came to give us

the good news that the medicine to reestablish normal heart rhythm had finally

worked! We never mentioned NAET to the nurse or doctor, but gave it full credit

for the now normal heart rhythm.

We were overjoyed that the heart catheterization, which had been planned for the next day was canceled and instead, the doctor discharged me from the hospital.

Five months later, I am a healthy 77 year old male, leading a full life and working part time - although week before last, I logged over 50 hours!

TYRIE C REYNOLDS MONROE, NC

SECTION K: IRRITABLE BOWEL SYNDROME (IBS)

June 23, 2008

Dr. Prince,

When I came to you a couple of years ago, I was suffering greatly from IBS. As I started the NAET treatments, I had a very open mind. I knew when medical science could do nothing *for me except to say, "You'll just have to learn to live with it", I was not going to accept that answer. I prayed that there was someone out there who could help. I was at my chiropractors' office in the waiting room and struck up a conversation with a young lady with her small daughter. She told me about NAET and how it helped her and her daughter. I called your office for an appointment. And boy am I glad I did!!! I went through the program and found I was allergic to EVERYTHING that I was tested for. I followed the procedure of staying away from the food I was being treated for, and found the next week, I was no longer allergic to that food. I didn't expect my stomach to react so quickly to the treatments but was pleased to realize that by the third treatment. I could eat foods that before would send me hunting a bathroom. My life style has changed because of these treatments and I am so grateful to you and your staff for the help I received. I only wish I had found out about you sooner. I recommend NAET for anyone, of any age, suffering from allergies or any illness.*

If you decide to give the treatments a try, you would be very surprised at the outcome. I have always been the type of person to believe if you don't try something yourself, you will never know if it could have helped or not. Thanks to you Dr. Prince, I am now a happier, healthier person today.

Sincerely,
Dianne Huffman   Maiden, NC

SECTION L: MOTION SICKNESS & POISON IVY

June 22, 2008

Dear Dr. Prince,

Before I began my NAET treatments, I had been seeing an alternative doctor in Asheville, NC. After a year or so of me seeing him once a month, he told me that he had done all he could do for me and the next step for me was a new treatment called NAET. He recommended I see you. He wanted me to see you because you were closer to me and he said you were very good.

I was so glad I did. For about ten years, I never saw a medical doctor. I came to see you for whatever was bothering me, from headache to cold. Whatever ailment I had, I wanted to see you.

I have two significant issues that you resolved for me that I'd like to share. There were many more...

I have always been highly allergic to poison ivy as a child and would get horrible cases of it even as an adult. I didn't have to touch it, just walk past it and I would break out. I am convinced I am completely cured of this. Not once have I had a reaction to poison ivy since you treated me.

Then the next biggie; my friends wanted to go on a cruise. Boy was I worried. I had never outgrown motion sickness, even riding in the front seat of a car I would still get nauseated. Sometimes I actually needed to stop the car and put my feet on the ground to stop the nausea. Well the cruise was a blast; I never felt the slightest nausea. What a great trip.

Thank you for all you have done for me.
Susan Croxton   Charlotte, NC

Note: For motions sickness, a surrogate lay face down on the table during treatment while holding the patient who was standing and weaving her head around simulating sea sickness. RMP

SECTION M: PAINT ALLERGY, ALSO MIGRAINE

5-12-08

Dear Dr. Prince,

After being a professional painter since 1961 I became allergic to paint and was having migraine headaches. After your NAET treatments for paint and migraine headaches I no longer have migraine headaches and I am longer allergic to paint.

Thank you very much.

John Baker   Glen Alpine, NC

SECTION N: CAT ALLERGIES

June 2008

Having experienced NAET treatments for about a year, I can attest that the outcome is positive and effective. I became an amazed believer after overcoming Cat Allergies. I would also add that it is very, very time consuming due to the touch ups of the original treatment. I have been a long time allergy sufferer and NAET has proved to be the most successful treatment.

P.B. Charlotte, NC

Note: Pat is right that NAET can be very time consuming. WE must not have stressed the fact that NAET is not a "quick fix." RMP

First let us apologize for editing some of these letters. We needed to make room for all that we could include and this meant paring down everywhere we could.

The heavy praise of these letters is somewhat embarrassing to us. Please consider giving the praise to the **NAET** treatments themselves. The only real negative I saw was a complaint about the length of time it takes and this is a very valid statement. "Rome wasn't built in a day," and better health takes time to achieve. We didn't get the way we are overnight either. We thank you all for your willing and generous participation in presenting the patients' views.

Wishing our participants and all our readers an improving journey into better health,

The authors.

INDEX

I

Ice cream 4, 47, 62, 84
Insomnia 24, 54, 59, 78. 87, 96

M

Milk 3, 5, 7, 14, 39, 43, 46-48,
54, 55, 59, 69. 81, 82, 88
Mold 74, 92
Multiple members of same
family 6, 7, 61-63, 71, 86-87
Muscle pain 32, 33

N

NCAAM 10, 11
Nuts 5, 7, 14, 38-40, 43, 44,
46-48, 55-57, 99

O

OCD 24

P

Paint 104
Peanuts 7, 14, 39-43, 46, 48.
53, 55-57, 99
Pizza 5, 84
Pollen 64, 74, 90
Poison Oak/Ivy 2, 92, 93, 102,
103
Psoriasis 73

R

Ragweed 75, 92
Red food dye 63

S

Shellfish 29, 98, 99
Shrimp 62, 92, 93, 98
Sinus problems 63
Spacey thoughts 61
Stomach problems 3, 59, 61,
62, 63, 71, 96, 102

T

Tomatoes 4, 5, 82, 88-90

V

Vomiting 25, 54, 59, 94

W

Water 66-68
Wheat 4, 5, 25, 26, 48, 69,
82, 85, 88

Y

Yogurt 5, 39, 47

For further information visit www.naet.com

Roberta Roberts
Mittman,
L. Ac, Dipl. Ac. M.S, PLLC

40 Park Ave, @ 36th st.
NY, NY 10046
       USA
(712) 686-0939

Printed in the United States
137811LV0000

for: Asthma + others